Let it Roll

Magic Moves to Conquer Your Aches & Pains and Create a Strong, Flexible Body

Fiona Naayen
B.App.Sc.Physio

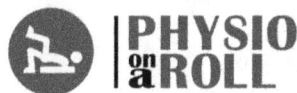

PHYSIO
on a ROLL

First published by Ultimate World Publishing 2021
Copyright © 2021 Fiona Naayen

ISBN

Paperback: 978-1-922497-72-7
Ebook: 978-1-922497-73-4

Cover design: Ultimate World Publishing
Layout and typesetting: Ultimate World Publishing
Editor: James Salmon

Ultimate World Publishing
Diamond Creek,
Victoria Australia 3089
www.writeabook.com.au

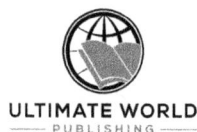

"If exercise could be packaged in a pill, it would be the single most widely prescribed and beneficial medicine in the nation."

Robert Butler

Disclaimer

While the advice and information in this book is believed to be accurate, there is risk involved and the author/publisher specifically disclaims any liability, loss or damage caused or alleged to be caused by this book and accepts no responsibility for inaccuracies/omissions in this book. This includes any adverse effects or consequences resulting from suggestions, exercises and advice in this book. Please do not use this book if you are not willing to assume the risk.

Contents

Introduction

Let it Roll!

This book is much more than an exercise program written by an Australian physiotherapist explaining and demonstrating safe, effective exercises with a foam roller. It is an accurate, contemporary book with useful information about all things exercise, pain, core and posture. It will show you how to perform exercises that focus on improving core strength, decreasing pain, and improving balance, flexibility and function. It will teach you how to use a foam roller safely and effectively, with graded exercises, from beginner to advanced. There are no fancy claims in this book – just the benefit of my experience and research and some great new ways to use a foam roller that you may not have thought of.

Physiotherapists are highly qualified health professionals who use advanced techniques and evidence-based care to assess, diagnose, treat and prevent a wide range of health conditions and movement disorders. So why have I, a physiotherapist with 28 years' experience, written this book about exercising with a foam roller? Well, simply, it is the culmination of many years of nagging by my clients (both past and present).

The foam roller features heavily in the clinic and the exercise classes I run. I find that those clients with pain tend to relax fully on the roller, "letting go" tight muscles. It helps with body and breath awareness. It makes it easier for people to activate and understand where their core muscles are and how to use them. I especially love the "ooohhs" and "aaahhhs" – the noises that people make when they lay on a long foam roller for the first time.

My clients have told me that they are after a book, video or photos to follow outside of the clinic when exercising at home or in the gym. They want the exercises they are doing in my classes or with me privately, on paper so that they can accurately show family and friends. And my stick figure drawings just weren't quite cutting it!

These clients are typically referred by friends, other physios or their medical practitioners to my exercise classes. They are hoping to ease back, neck, knee, hip or shoulder pain mostly after they've had hands-on treatment or because they are sick of hands-on treatment failing to settle their "niggles". Many sit at a desk for hours each day. Some are osteoporotic. Others have fallen, been in a car accident or tweaked something playing golf. Often, exercise is not a priority. Or exercise is not seen as an option because they are fearful of moving in case their pain is aggravated. All of these clients, however, want to feel better. To eliminate pain. To improve their core strength, their mobility and feel fitter, stronger and leaner. They want to go about their daily life without pain and live well.......... and age well.

I have found that using a foam roller facilitates all of this.

I have searched for an up-to-date, comprehensive, safe and easy to follow foam roller resource for my clients to use outside of the clinic. Online or in print. But it does not appear to exist. If you Google "foam roller exercises" or look on Instagram you will find that other exercise professionals confine the roller to myofascial and muscle releases. Or they feature advanced Pilates routines that are set at a level far too complex for the average person to follow – especially the average person with a neck or lower back issue. Other publications lack detailed explanations or make wild claims about the foam roller's magical abilities (they do not dissolve cellulite or "melt" fascia by the way!)

So, I created a website called **Physio on a Roll** and started photographing, videoing and adding detailed explanations and tips to the photos. This has now morphed into this book.

Now, the evidence for foam rollers is complex. There is not a lot of research at this point in time and much of it is flawed. However, the reliable research that does exist (and my own experience over many years) points to the fact that using a foam roller has benefits. It helps people manage stress, helps them to relax and improves their joint proprioception (your ability to tell where your joint is in space). Anecdotally, people feel better using a roller. And importantly, there are no negatives [1][2][28].

What we do know is that exercise and movement in general can be amongst the most powerful ways to reduce and improve pain. We also now know that specific exercise programs designed to improve strength and endurance can decrease pain by around 60% [3].

A recent Sydney University study found that 7/10 people with low back pain will have another episode within a year. Researchers found that the only known way to prevent this reoccurrence was a prolonged exercise program of six months or more [4].

As well as strengthening bone and muscles, exercise can also promote healing, prevent disease, and improve mood and mental health. Exercising increases lifespan, brain function and improves your quality of life [5]. It also makes you look better naked!

My hope with this book is to help you know why you are performing particular exercises. You will learn how exercise can help you manage your specific issue and how to exercise at an appropriate level. I encourage you to read the theory sections at the beginning of this book to understand these concepts and to be honest about where you need to start.

As an exercise tool, the foam roller is portable, practical and ideal for all ages and fitness levels to use. I hope to encourage greater use of the humble foam roller and believe it should have a place in your office or lounge room. Use your roller with this book as a guide and roll often, move well and improve your health.

Roll, Move, Improve!

CHAPTER 1

Why roll? The top 11 reasons for including a roller in your workout

So why should you foam roll?

1. **To figure out where your core muscles are and what they do –** the foam roller is a long, cylindrical piece of firm-ish foam. When you lie on it or stand on it, you will wobble. Your body is supported on an essentially unstable surface and will be searching for stability. With the correct instruction*, the roller can help you to locate and activate your core muscles. These core muscles work together

---

* the correct instructions will help you to minimise compensations and guide you to movement that is smooth and effortless.

to support your spine and allow your limbs to move. See the next chapter for more insight into your core.

2. **Challenge your balance** – once again, the roller's inherent instability will enhance your balance reactions whether you lie on it, stand on it or incorporate it into lunges and lifts. We know that the more we challenge our balance the better chance we have of improving it (6). We also know that balance control declines with age (especially after the age of 50 years) and that we need to do around an hour of balance training each week to maintain our balance (7), and more if we want to improve it. Enhancing your balance reactions is also beneficial on the sporting field when you are required to respond and move quickly.

Impaired balance is a major risk factor for falls amongst older adults (8).

3. **Mindfulness** – yes, a bit of an overused term of late but really all we are talking about when we reference "mindfulness" is the ability to think, focus and be present with what you are doing. The roller encourages mindful movement as you have to think and be aware when performing your very skill-based exercises. Otherwise, if you are lying on the roller, you may fall off!

Making this even more important is that we know that you may achieve more muscle fibre recruitment when you think about what you are doing (9).

4. **Better breathing** – when exercising on a long foam roller, your slow, thoughtful and controlled movements will make you much more aware of your breathing. You will start to appreciate how important your breathing is to your ability to activate your core and how better breathing can contribute to muscle relaxation around your neck and spine. As a physio, I have found the roller, when laid on top of, to be an invaluable tool in helping people learn about diaphragmatic breathing. More on this in the next chapter.

5. **Postural awareness** – there is no "perfect posture", but the foam roller can help to create a better posture for most people. Posture is another topic tackled in a little more depth in the following chapter. Suffice to say that when using a

roller your posture is enhanced because the foam roller helps you to learn how to switch off overactive, tight and sore muscle groups. You will have a better chance of using your deeper muscles, particularly in your neck. Many of the exercises in this book encourage you to be aware of where your neck and spine are in space when you are exercising. You will also progress your understanding of your core and the differences between each side of your body.

6. **Increased mobility** – mobility refers to your active range of motion. A lot of the exercises that you will do with a roller will encourage you to move through a full range of movement through your joints, sometimes under load or with resistance. Moving actively through this range helps to build your mobility and also build strength and stability.

The roller also helps to switch off unwanted muscle activity. An example that comes to mind is the shoulder's range of motion in supine (lying on your back with your face and torso facing up) on a roller. If we focus on the shoulder we can "let go" of the large neck muscles that can dominate shoulder function and unnecessarily lift the shoulder towards the ear.

7. **Increased flexibility** – flexibility refers to the passive range of motion at a given joint. Rolling out your muscles will help you to feel relaxed and "lengthened" and enhance your flexibility. It is what most people use their foam roller for. There is some debate about the roller's ability to "release fascia" but the general consensus is that people who foam roll after exercise feel better and it improves joint proprioception (which is the ability to tell where your joint is in space) (1)(2). Importantly, there are no negative effects of using a foam roller to improve flexibility.

8. **Increased variety and challenge to an existing workout** – now, you could do your bench press, flys and triceps exercises lying on a bench. But do them on a long foam roller and it takes your workout to a whole new level! You can feel your core contracting as you have to maintain your position on the roller and move your weights. Similarly, when doing a push up on the roller on the floor, the wobbles on the roller combined with using your body weight as resistance really challenges your core.

The inherent instability as described before primes your core, especially if you do unilateral exercises. You do want to include weights and resistance in your workout with a roller as the benefits are many and are discussed at length in the following chapter.

9. **Inexpensive –** as a piece of exercise equipment, the roller is a relatively inexpensive item given the great variety of exercises that it can be used for. Look for a very dense EVA roller that won't distort or bend. If you go for a covered foam roller, such as the *Physio on a Roll* design featured in this book then it will survive dents and gouges as well and should last for years.

10. **Practical –** even the average long foam roller at 90cm x 15cm x 15cm is very lightweight and portable. It does not take up too much space. It fits easily under a bed or behind a door. It is preferable that you don't hide it away though, because out of sight generally means out of mind and you should be trying to use your roller every day.

11. **Accessible for everybody –** anybody, regardless of age, body type, activity level (beginner or athlete), stress level, occupation, condition or symptom can exercise with a foam roller. I have clients well into their 80s using a foam roller post knee and hip replacements. I also have elite-level basketballers and rowers using a roller to train their core and add challenge to balance exercises.

CHAPTER 2

Drumroll......Before you roll

"Your present circumstances don't determine where you can go; they merely determine where you start."

Nido Qubein

I encourage you to read through this chapter fully so that you understand some of the theory around exercise and related concepts such as your core, pain and neuromuscular training. This will help you to be honest about where you need to start.

Before you exercise

As a physiotherapist, before a new client begins any treatment or exercise program I am required to ask them to fill in a form outlining their health history. Read through the statements below and if any of them apply to you then I suggest that you speak to your doctor before you start exercising.

1. Your chest hurts when you do physical activity.
2. Your doctor has said that you have a heart condition and should only do physical activity recommended by a doctor.
3. In the past month you have experienced chest pain when you were not doing any physical activity.
4. You suffer from loss of balance due to dizzy spells (vertigo) or you are prone to fainting.
5. You are on medication for high blood pressure or a heart condition.
6. You have a severe scoliosis or severe kyphosis (spinal curvatures).
7. You have had a recent fracture or cancer diagnosis*.
8. You have been diagnosed as osteoporotic**.
9. You are at all unsure about using a foam roller for exercising.

If any of these statements do apply to you, it does not necessarily mean that you cannot do the exercises. It only flags that you should speak to your doctor prior to starting.

Precautions: Generally, whenever you start a new exercise regime, especially if you have not exercised for some time, it is wise to start slowly and with the basics.

If you experience pain performing any of the exercises featured in this book...........
STOP. Read through the "tips" that accompany the exercise instructions. Check your technique and execution of the exercise. Watch the exercise video online, via the Physio on a Roll website. If there is still pain when you perform the move again, *try an easier option from the menu* or omit it from your routine. *In general,* all your roller exercises should be performed *without back or neck pain*. The basic roller exercises are designed to help you to activate your deep stabilising muscles. These deep muscles are switched on at a low-level of muscle contraction.

---

* In most cases, exercise is now being used as adjunct to cancer treatment (10)(29).

** Exercise and bone maintenance are inextricably linked (11).

As such, all the roller exercises should be able to be performed in a pain-free manner. When lying on the roller you can use a pillow for support at your neck, at least initially, so that the chosen exercise can be performed without pain.

If you find that the pressure of the roller is uncomfortable, drape a thick towel over the roller. Alternatively, choose a less dense roller on which to perform your exercises and then progress to a harder/denser roller as you are able. Please note that you can also attempt almost all of the beginner exercises on the floor without a roller. Simply master the floor position and then progress onto a roller.

Let's talk a little more about pain

In general, our thinking about pain and how we "treat" it has changed over the last decade. We know that the human body is strong, resilient and able to adapt. It is rare to cause permanent injury to your body (12).

Here are 9 facts that every person needs to know about pain (12,13):

- Pain is far more complex than we ever imagined.
- Pain is an experience, not a sensation – it is also a signal, not a problem.
- Your pain is real.
- Pain does not equal tissue damage – for example, having a sore wrist does not usually mean that your wrist is damaged. It may indicate that it is hypersensitive, i.e. the pain at the wrist is made to feel worse or sensitised by muscle tension. Typically this occurs because you are not using your wrist or are moving it awkwardly, are adopting different postures, or are suffering from a lack of sleep, stress, anxiety or simply worrying about your wrist. Often wrist soreness is due to a minor strain that can be painful but will heal on its own. Sleeping well and staying physically active will substantially improve your rate of recovery. Worrying may actually have the undesired effect of increasing pain due to the undivided attention towards the sensation of pain. This holds true with back and neck pain as well.

- The words we use when we talk about pain have the power to make pain better or worse.
- Imaging, such as X-rays, ultrasounds and MRIs have the power to make your pain better or worse. The scan results need to be put into perspective as many of the changes that are seen and reported on are often a normal part of the aging process – just like grey hair, wrinkles and wisdom! Often asymptomatic people of the same age will have a similar or worse appearance on a scan.
- Movement can be among the most powerful ways to improve pain. The human body gets stronger with movement. If we try to avoid movement or move with fear you can actually make pain worse. We need to remember that MOTION IS LOTION. Moving might be uncomfortable initially, but as you continue to move it will improve. Movement helps the body to heal and boosts the immune system. Avoiding movement can lead to an increase in disability and further loss of wellbeing.
- To know pain = to know gain. As a physio I work on S.M.A.R.T* plans that help people manage their pain by modifying their work or swapping a sport or exercise.
- You can still live well with pain. Pain flare-ups can happen but they will settle, as they have done in the past.

Benefits of exercise

The scientific evidence demonstrating the positive effects of exercise on the human body is indisputable. In most adults, the benefits of exercise far outweigh the risks. Being physically active:

- lowers blood pressure.
- improves the way the body processes blood lipids and blood sugar.
- increases bone density.
- has positive effects on articular cartilage (see p.20).

---

* S.M.A.R.T = Specific, Measurable, Achievable, Realistic and Timely

- decreases fatigue, so that the body becomes more efficient and requires less energy to do the same amount of work.
- improves mood through the release of endorphins and serotonin.
- prevents many other chronic diseases. Being inactive actually increases the risk of at least 35 chronic diseases (14).

Physical activity recommendations

In Australia, it's recommended that adults should complete around 150 minutes of moderate exercise or 75 minutes of vigorous exercise per week (40).

You should exercise at an intensity where you feel slightly short of breath or you start sweating. To improve your physical fitness you need to exercise at 60% of your max heart rate (220 - age). For most adults, an exercise program that includes aerobic, resistance, neuromotor/neuromuscular and flexibility exercises will improve and maintain physical fitness and health.

For many of us though, physical restrictions or injuries and particularly pain limit our ability and willingness to participate in exercise. Exercise programs such as those in *Let it Roll* can help to ease your aches and pains and improve your strength and mobility so that you can build your capacity to be active and achieve these physical activity goals.

As a physiotherapist, I am experienced at using exercise as therapy, prescribing therapeutic exercises to correct movement impairments, reduce pain and restore muscular and skeletal function. The types of exercise physios prescribe fall into 4 main groups, which I will discuss in greater detail below:

1. Resistance exercises, also known as strength training
2. Neuromuscular exercises that work to improve the brain to muscle connection
3. Flexibility exercises achieved through stretching and movement
4. Balance and coordination exercises that focus on maintaining an individual's centre of gravity.

Resistance exercise

Resistance exercise is also known as weight or strength training. It involves moving parts of your body against some kind of resistance, like weights, resistance bands, weight machines, or even your own body weight (such as in a push-up or squat).

Why should you do resistance exercise?

Resistance exercise helps to build stronger muscles. It also strengthens your bones and joints, reducing your chance of injury and improving your balance and posture, and can even boost your metabolism, affecting insulin levels and helping with dementia (15).

Incorporating resistance training into your exercise routine is very important, especially as you age. From around your 40s you begin to lose muscle mass and strength in a process known as age-related sarcopenia. Muscles shrink. Fat accumulates. At 50, physically inactive people will lose 1-2% of their muscle mass each year and 10% or more per decade. Strength declines twice as fast as muscle mass and power declines even faster than strength. Even if you are active, you'll still have some muscle loss. The more muscle mass you have at your peak, the more you will have left as age takes its toll. Research also shows that you can add size and strength at any age and that the less you have pushed yourself to get where you are now, the more potential you have to improve (16).

NB. The primary treatment for sarcopenia is exercise, specifically resistance training.

So how do you build muscle?

When you exercise, as long as it requires effort and the effort produces fatigue and you feel those fatigued muscles, then you will end up with stronger and better developed muscles. Challenging your muscles in a workout creates micro tears and, to put it simply, unleashes a cascade of chemical signals and responses. One of those signals activates satellite cells on the outside of the muscle fibres. These satellite cells attempt to repair the micro damage by joining together and, as a result, increase the size of the muscle fibre.

Resistance training also stimulates your body to release growth hormone from your pituitary gland. How much is released depends on the intensity of the exercise you've done. Growth hormone in turn triggers your metabolism and helps to turn amino acids into protein to grow or "bulk" up your muscles. It is worth noting that men and women build muscles differently due to the role testosterone plays in muscle development. While both sexes have testosterone in their bodies, men have more of this hormone. However, studies have shown that both men and women have similar responses to strength training. It goes without saying that adequate hydration, sleep, rest and a good diet also contribute to muscle development.

A note on muscle soreness: We know that when we are trying to build muscle we are also damaging it – micro tears happen, as explained above, and the body repairs that damage, adding another layer of support or more muscle.

The body's response to the tearing or damage is to flood the area with specialist repair cells and to trigger pain receptors. So, muscle soreness, which usually presents a day or two after intense exercise (known as delayed onset muscle soreness or DOMS) is not caused by the micro damage but is related to the body's inflammatory response to it. DOMS can strike any time that the *frequency, duration* or *intensity* of your workout is increased. This is generally positive, especially if your aim is to improve strength, stamina, speed or size. It indicates that your body is adapting to meet the increased physical demands placed upon it. If you are trying to improve strength for example, you need to break down some of your existing muscle structure to create bigger, stronger and more capable muscles going forward.

The signature symptoms of DOMS – extreme or atypical soreness, joint stiffness and tenderness – tend to surface 12-24 hours post-activity. DOMS may worsen for up to 72 hours post-activity. You can help yourself during this period of discomfort by staying active, even though it may feel like the last thing you want to do. You are more likely to get positive adaptive changes in the structure of your muscles by continuing to exercise gently. Try not to give yourself time off. It is also important to stay hydrated and you can use ice to ease pain, especially for the first 24-48 hours.

After *Let it Roll* workouts you may feel a little sore but should not have trouble walking downstairs!

Rollers and DOMS: Strategic use of a foam roller can also be a great way to ease DOMS. Rolling can improve the blood circulation to the affected area. This aids in the removal of the by-products of the inflammatory response (see the Roll and Release Chapter 7 for specific exercises to ease DOMS).

Neuromuscular exercise

The brain, nervous system and muscles work together to allow you to perform a movement or skill. *Ideally*, in the body, the muscles that stabilise the joints work in balance with the muscles that move the joints. This produces smooth and efficient movement, minimal wear and tear on the joints, and as a result, less likelihood of pain. If a joint has this "balance", you can say that you have good *motor control.*

Sometimes this movement comes naturally, such as using your legs to walk. But often we have to learn how to do a movement or perform a skill. Think back to when you first learnt to ride a bike. Initially it was challenging and unnatural. Practice improved your skills and it became something that you could do without thinking about it.

The brain to muscle connection can be weakened or damaged through an injury or poor movement patterns. Poor movement patterns can then create muscle imbalances that become poor movement habits. This can cause pain.

Put simply, sometimes some of our muscles don't work enough and other muscles are overactive. Our hip flexors and our glutes (bottom muscles) are great examples. Sitting on our bottoms all day can encourage short/tight hip or psoas muscles and weak, ineffectual gluteals. Muscle imbalances like these are often associated with our increasingly sedentary lifestyles. These imbalanced muscles will continue to work inefficiently and often painfully until we *retrain the brain.*

Regular neuromuscular activation exercises can help to improve the brain and muscle connection and help you to gain better control over your muscles, improve muscle strength, and improve your balance and joint control. As your muscles work better together you will achieve more from your workouts and move more fluently and functionally throughout your day-to-day life.

How do I improve my motor control?

Many years of research has demonstrated that we can correct poor movement patterns. We just need to start simply and repeat better patterns over and over again, until the better movement pattern becomes automatic.

Let it Roll uses a motor control approach to initially teach you how to gain control of the correct muscles in simple postures, doing simple movements while breathing normally.

You then progress by adopting more challenging and complex postures and by adding resistance such as weights and bands. Many exercises are then given a further functional component. This means that the prescribed exercise aims to train your muscles to work together and simulate a real-world activity, or resemble a common movement you do every day or may perform in sport. Often the upper and lower body work together at the same time so many of the intermediate and advanced exercises in *Let it Roll* reflect this. For example, leaning over a sink to spit out your toothpaste is similar to a "forward lean" or hip hinge exercise.

Flexibility exercise

Flexibility refers to the passive range of motion at a given joint. Stretching is different to flexibility and can lead to an increase in flexibility. Do you often feel tight or stiff? The need to stretch often arises because a muscle gets tight. Tight muscles are almost always strong muscles. Our bodies and brains are very clever and when another muscle fails, the strong muscle comes in to save the day. The strong muscles are asked to do their normal job and then make up for another one not pulling its weight. The strong muscles sometimes do too much and get tight. This is a result of a breakdown in our movement patterns or sometimes motor control. We need to learn why you are getting tight and how to get that normal movement back.

Balance exercise

Balance is the ability to control your body's position, whether stationary (e.g. in a complex yoga pose) or while moving (e.g. walking down stairs).

It is a complex skill that involves continuous interaction between:

- the brain – your brain asks your body "where am I?"
- the eyes – they tell your brain how well you are aligned vertically and horizontally (using reference points such as trees, vertical walls).
- the fluid filled canals in the inner ear – which sense head movement, telling you whether you are leaning or swaying.
- your muscles, tendons and ligaments – think glutes and especially your legs and ankles, which sense how much tension is pulling on them, giving you clues about your position in space.
- your feet – they sense the pressure of your body weight.

Balance is a "use it or lose it" kind of thing. If you don't practice, the coordination between these body parts can deteriorate over time, making it harder for you to stay upright and making you predisposed to injury (17).

Our vision tends to offer quick and easy information about our position in space and most of the time this is what we rely on, ignoring the information from the inner ear and legs. When it is dark or there are lots of moving objects in sight, the brain relies on fast and accurate information from the inner ear and legs (rather than our eyes). But if the brain has not been paying much attention to these body parts, then it becomes slow at processing their information, and our balance is poor as a result.

When you have good balance, you have an improved ability to quickly adapt to changes in body position, adjusting on the fly to unexpected variations. Your brain is able to continuously make quick decisions, in the background, and send very fast signals to our muscles to control our balance, even when we are pre-occupied.

There is evidence to show that balance improves when using a time-based or repetition-style exercise program (7).

Osteoarthritis

There is a lot of fear and misunderstanding about exercising with osteoarthritis (OA). Often people have been advised that rest and avoidance of exercise is best. Sometimes people become fearful of movement, assuming that they will cause more damage to their joint if they experience pain with movement.

There is now an increasing amount of quality research (18) that shows that exercise is safe and can significantly reduce pain and disability in those people suffering with OA (see next page).

In fact, any type of exercise, whether that be walking or strength training, has proved to be effective for pain relief. Specific exercises, particularly neuromuscular exercises (such as those detailed in this book) have been shown to increase muscle strength and endurance and improve stability and trust in the affected joint. Research also points to the fact that the pain people experience is more related to decreasing muscle strength (especially with knee OA and quad strength) than the changes in the joints that may be evident on their X-ray scans (19).

Neuromuscular exercises often simulate the activities that you perform as part of your everyday life. Learning how to move well and load your joints through moderate doses of exercise can positively influence cartilage health and reduce the risk of developing OA. We also know that exercise helps with weight loss and enhancing mood, which also benefits your joints and decreases pain perception.

Osteoarthritis

Osteoarthritis (OA) is a common joint disease and is an accepted reason for people not being active as they age. The three joints *most often* affected by OA are the knee, hip and hands, but any joint in the body covered with articular cartilage can be affected.

Synovial joint

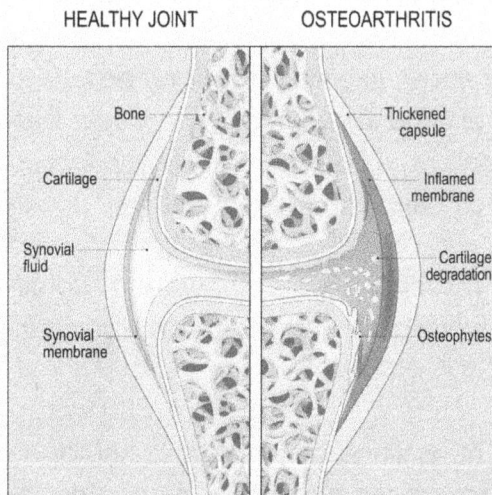

HEALTHY JOINT   OSTEOARTHRITIS

Bone
Cartilage
Synovial fluid
Synovial membrane

Thickened capsule
Inflamed membrane
Cartilage degradation
Osteophytes

Around 5% of people between 35 and 54 years of age have OA. Many of these folk have injured their joint earlier in life. Women are more likely to have OA than men and more often it is in their knees and hands. OA often has a hereditary component and approximately 1/3 of the population between the ages of 50 and 70 years have problems related to OA. This percentage increases as we age (19).

Osteoarthritis affects the whole joint but most of all it affects the *articular cartilage* (which is the cartilage covering the ends of the bones). Articular cartilage is solid but flexible, absorbing shock and spreading loads over its surface. It has no blood supply or pain sensors (so it cannot "hurt"). The cartilage instead relies on the movement of water in and out of it to feed it and keep it clean. Think of the cartilage as a wet sponge. When a load is applied, fluid is forced out. When the load is removed, fluid is sucked back in. When we walk, for example, our body weight and gravity press down on the cartilage in our knee, pushing out fluid. When we aren't weight bearing on that leg, the fluid is sucked back in.

With OA there is a breakdown in this transportation of water in and out of the cartilage. More often than not this is due to not enough water being squeezed out of cartilage – which means that waste products are not removed and the cartilage's environment becomes a bit toxic. This then begins a chemical cascade and, to put it simply, begins to degrade the cartilage. The cartilage becomes thin, it may crack and can even disappear altogether. Bones can then start to rub against each other. This is OA – when there is more degeneration than regeneration of the cartilage. OA is irreversible, but the symptoms (pain, stiffness, swelling, decreased range of motion) can be reduced and even disappear.

So exercise and joint loading is essential for cartilage health. It is often too little loading rather than too much that is the culprit! Cartilage needs a certain amount of load to regenerate. This is why healthy loads need to be applied to joints for cartilage recovery.

Rest is rust, motion is lotion. It is not "wear and tear", but better to think of it as "load and adapt".

Osteoporosis

Osteoporosis literally means porous bone and is characterised by low bone mass and poor bone quality. Osteoporosis prevalence increases with age, but usually has no symptoms until a fracture occurs. *Osteopenia* is when your bones are weaker than normal but they are not likely to break easily, unlike osteoporosis.

Exercise and bone maintenance are inextricably linked. Exercise helps to build and maintain strong bones and prevent falls and fractures by improving balance, co-ordination, muscle strength and agility. To have an effect on bone and maximise bone adaptation, exercise needs to be regular (at least 3x/week), progressive (becomes more challenging over time) and fairly vigorous, varied and performed in short intense bursts. The exercise should be weight-bearing (i.e. performed whilst on your feet) and strength enhancing. High impact activities such as jogging, jumping and rope skipping are more stimulating to bone cells than sustained, low impact activity such as walking. Novel forces, such as changing directions and different heights of jumps are more stimulating than repetitive force patterns. Exercising in short bouts with rest periods seems to be more effective than continuous, long periods of exercise. Continuous progression is the most critical element of the exercise prescription for bone health. If the progression stops, so does the adaptation in the bone and muscle (20)(30).

Osteoporosis explained

Bone is divided into cancellous (or trabecular) bone and cortical bone. Cancellous bone is more metabolically active and is formed by interconnecting latticework. Cancellous bone is surrounded by the less delicate cortical bone. Bone is remodelled (or turned over) throughout adult life by discrete remodelling units of osteoclasts (cells that resorb bone) and osteoblasts (cells that lay down new bone).

As we age (especially after 50 years), the volume of bone resorbed is greater than the volume formed in each remodelling unit. This process accelerates during menopause. This is because decreasing oestrogen levels enhances the rate of bone resolution. This continues in old age (i.e. over 70 years of age). Your family history, low calcium and vitamin D levels increase your risk of becoming osteoporotic. Similarly, a medical history of hormonal and metabolic factors such as - *in women:* delayed puberty, early menopause, *in men:* low testosterone – can elevate your risk. Thyroid conditions, conditions leading to malabsorption (e.g. coeliac disease), chronic diseases such as liver or kidney disease and taking certain medications – e.g. corticosteroids (commonly used for asthma, rheumatoid arthritis) – increase your risk of brittle bones. Lifestyle factors such as low levels of physical activity, smoking, excessive alcohol intake and being over or under weight are also known risk factors.

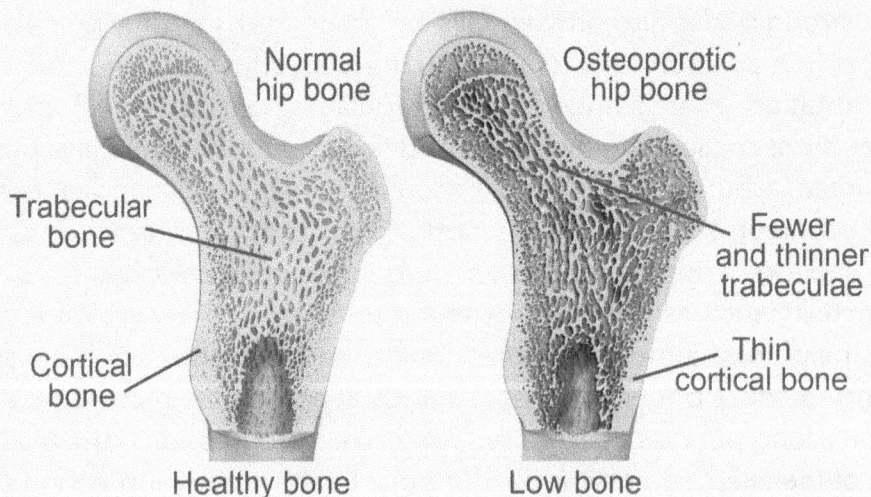

Normal hip bone

Osteoporotic hip bone

Trabecular bone

Fewer and thinner trabeculae

Cortical bone

Thin cortical bone

Healthy bone

Low bone

Posture

Firstly, what is posture? It basically refers to the position of our body in space – but it is a lot more complicated than we previously thought.

Posture is a product of spinal reflexes and some extra "tweaking" in your brain, all of which occurs without the involvement of your conscious thought or attention. While you can consciously change your posture (e.g. trying not to slump in a chair with no back support) you will generally revert back to the unconscious and reflex control pattern when your mind wanders. Importantly, there is no perfect posture. We all have very differently built bodies and studies show that our posture is highly individual (21). In fact, posture will vary within an individual depending on a whole host of different factors, including our mood, the load, our tolerance and capacity, and the length of time spent in a position.

Your posture, or how you hold your body, is part of the "stress" on tissues, but there are many variables other than posture that influence injuries. As a result, we no longer think of posture as good or bad.

While "poor" posture, for example being slumped over a desk for prolonged periods, is not ideal for feeling good, neither is sitting bolt upright. We could all probably think of a person who has a "nice" posture who is in terrible pain as well as a person with "lousy" posture with no pain. The fact is that recent research (22) shows that no one posture is perfect. Our body and particularly our spines are strong and stable and have an amazing ability to adapt and are also capable of all sorts of great things. A specific posture doesn't necessarily correlate to pain. Of more importance is regular movement and changing positions often to remain pain free. "Motion is lotion." Morgan Freeman put it quite succinctly when he said, "Your best posture is your next posture".

So when we talk about improving our posture we perhaps need to rephrase it and consider increasing our "postural fitness".

Breathing

Breathing is one of the most natural and automatic processes in the body. We breathe to deliver oxygen to the body and when we are exercising, we need a smooth and efficient breath to deliver more oxygen to the working muscles. The more efficiently that you deliver this oxygen to your muscles, the harder and more effectively you can exercise. Whether you are exercising or at rest, diaphragmatic breathing is the most efficient and effective method of breathing.

As a physiotherapist, I see lots of people with neck, shoulder and back pain. Often they are "upper chest" breathers. That means that when they breathe, they use their neck and shoulder muscles to assist their breathing. Why? Our busy, modern life stops us breathing well. If we are stressed, we often take small, quick breaths. Tight-fitting clothes, ill-fitting bras, and the desire to look thinner (and therefore suck your tummy in) all affect diaphragmatic breathing. Sitting for long periods at a desk, hunched over, makes it easier to use the neck and shoulders to breathe, but will add to neck pain when those muscles fatigue.

If you can learn to "breathe into your diaphragm" (the large muscle located between your chest and tummy) you can engage your core effectively and let the neck, shoulders and back muscles relax. You might also find you feel calmer because your parasympathetic nervous system is activated, setting up a "rest and digest" response which opposes the "flight or fight" response of the sympathetic nervous system. There is some evidence to show that slow, controlled diaphragmatic breathing can reduce the levels of cortisol (the stress hormone) in the saliva and affect the levels of another hormone, noradrenaline, in the brain (23)(47).

Diaphragmatic breathing – a guide

The first step to improving your breathing is to become aware of it. An easy method is to lie in supine with one hand on your tummy and the other on your chest. As you breathe in you want to feel your tummy rise and as you breathe out your tummy should fall. The hand on your chest should not move much at all.

Another way to visualise breathing is to think of a paper lantern. The diaphragm is the top of the lantern, your abdominal muscles make up the front and sides, the back muscles are the rear and your pelvic floor (PF) is the underside of the lantern. As you breathe in and air fills your lungs, the top of the lantern drops down and the lantern becomes floppy. As you breathe out the top and bottom of the lantern rises and the lantern walls become tightened. If we relate that to your core, we should breathe out when we move to help to engage the abdominal and PF muscles more efficiently.

It is important to realise that diaphragmatic breathing can be intuitive for some people but can take time for others to learn. But DON'T get hung up with your breathing during exercise. Just breathe. It will improve with practice.

Discovering the right pairing of your breath with each movement is a personal journey. In general, you should be breathing in at the beginning of a movement and breathing out as you move.

With strength training, breathing out during the concentric phase (the phase where you overcome gravity, for example the upward part of a push-up) of the exercise can help you to lift more weight as you create core pressure that stabilises your spine.

During mobility focused exercises such as Pilates and yoga, longer, deeper breathing will help you to better access your range of motion. You can often achieve a bigger stretch/range with a repeated exhalation.

With aerobic exercises, you should try to establish a consistent breathing pattern. That means even, measured breaths rather than short, shallow breaths. This will ensure that your working muscles receive the oxygen that they need.

It is worth noting that ideally you want to breathe through the nose, as your nasal passages help to humidify the air and filter out pollution, allergens and bacteria before they travel to your lungs. However, if you are exercising heavily you cannot take in as much air as needed through your nose, which is why people tend to mouth breathe during intense exercise.

Core

Your core is the area between your hips and your shoulders. It is the link between your limbs and your trunk and refers to the many abdominal, lower back and hip muscles that surround your spine and keep your trunk upright. It includes transversus abdominus, the internal and external obliques, rectus abdominus, erector spinae, multifidus, the diaphragm, the pelvic floor, longissimus, quadratus lumborum and the glutes. I like to include the gluteal muscles because they have such an important part to play in stability and movement.

Your core is involved in everything that you do. The core muscles align your spine, ribs and pelvis and stabilise your spine while your limbs move; i.e. your limb muscles create motion while the trunk muscles primarily stop motion.

Your core muscles also allow you to move your spine and torso forwards (flexion), backwards (extension), and side to side (lateral flexion) as well as to rotate. So if you utilise these movements of flexion, extension, lateral flexion and rotation in your exercises as well as compound movements, like squats, presses and pulls, you will create a well-rounded exercise program that will engage and improve your core.

And what about core exercises?

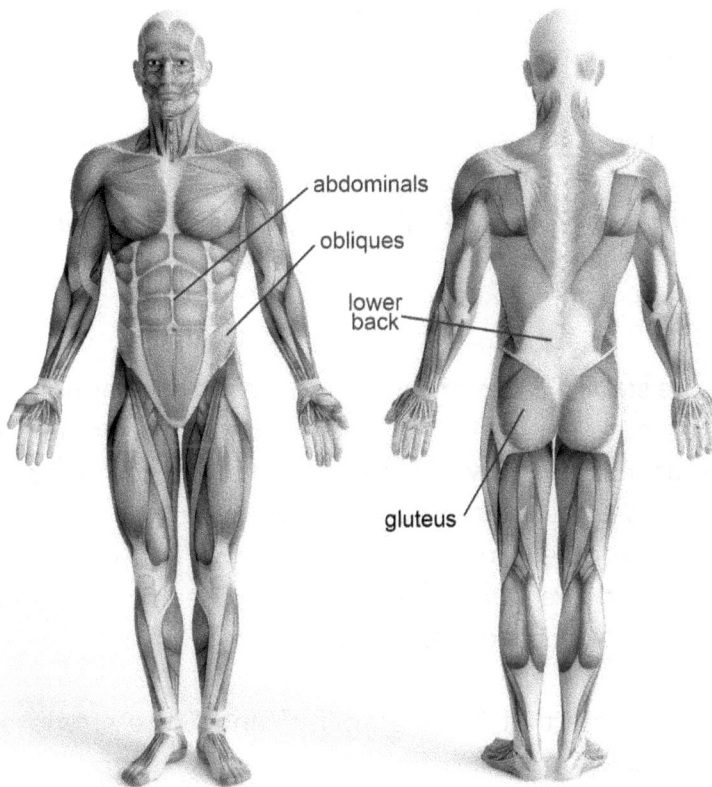

abdominals
obliques
lower back
gluteus

You could probably call any exercise in which the body is not being supported a core exercise. In a push-up, for example, the back and abdominal muscles must contract to keep the spine straight as you use your shoulder girdle and chest to lower the body. In another example, doing a single arm fly with a weight on a foam roller requires you to activate muscles in the stomach, spine, hips and pelvis to balance and support the body while the arm moves out to the side.

The point of core exercises is to train the many large and small muscles that help to move and support the spinal column and pelvis. These muscles may then have an improved ability to efficiently move the body when forces are applied to it (like bending, reaching and twisting) during the simple tasks you do in everyday life. The benefit is that this can then hopefully minimise injury. The last thing you want is to hurt your back when you bend down to pick up your child or grandchild.

If your core muscles are working well then there is less chance of sustaining an injury from an everyday task.

Core exercises can and should be incorporated into every workout you perform. And, if you are training all the major body areas such as your chest, back, shoulders and legs regularly, then your core will more than likely be being trained too.

What is "core stability"?

In the 1990's "core stability" became very trendy. The assumption was that certain muscles were far more important for stabilisation of the spine than others, i.e. if your transversus abdominus was weak it could lead to back pain. It was also thought that the core muscles were a unique group of muscles that worked independently of the other trunk muscles. We now know that there is *"strong evidence to show that core stabilisation exercises are no more effective than any other form of active exercise in the long term"* (24).

We also now appreciate that "core stability" and "core strength" are not the same. We should really be talking about *core motor control.*

So what does "core motor control" mean?

Greg Dea and Rod Harris (25) have summarised it succinctly; *"Movement can be viewed as being clean and easy or dirty and difficult and we (as physios) step in to correct when it becomes dirty and difficult".*

As an example, if you have to think about your core, every time, *before* you bend over to pick a toy up off the floor, something is wrong. The problem is that the instant you get distracted you forget about your core. So just training conscious core control is not ideal but **it is useful initially.** Core motor control is actually reflex driven, not consciously driven. We have to leave our brain to do what it does so well in a way that we could never coach. It goes back to the same concept I discussed with neuromuscular exercises with brain-to-muscle connection – the brain-to-muscle connection can be weakened or damaged through an injury or poor movement patterns. Poor movement patterns can then create imbalances that become poor movement habits, and this can cause pain.

So as a physio, my role is to decrease any pain and mobility restrictions that you may have so that the exercises I give you can challenge your ability to use that reflex. I then look at how you perform that exercise and assess if it is "clean and easy" or "dirty and difficult". If it is deemed "dirty and difficult", then I need to cue the processing occurring, i.e. the timing and sequencing, so that it is organised in a way that produces a better movement.......so that the movement becomes "clean and easy".

So where does that leave us?

If you want to train your core, just exercise. If you have pain, just move. You may need *guidance at first* to improve your core motor control so that the quality of your movement becomes "clean and easy". But ultimately, you want your core to fire automatically.

If you don't change "dirty and difficult" movement then you are working harder and harder each time you repeat the movement. You are inefficient. Fatigue will probably come on sooner and you will increase your risk of injury.

Basic core activation

If you are returning to exercise after an injury or still have pain, you can't expect to launch into planks and squats successfully without learning some basics. Sometimes it can help if you think about your core as being like an onion. There are many layers. All the layers bind and weave and work together to produce efficient movement, and your core is involved with everything that you do.

As an example, when lifting a weight with your right arm, in front of your body, the muscles of the core work together well to support the spine. You ***should automatically*** gently lift the pelvic floor muscles and draw the abdominal and back muscles in a little to support the spine, while your breathing is normal and easy. The ***core*** muscles are all engaged gently as you lift the weight out in front of the body and then return, and then the core muscles relax. This sometimes isn't an automatic response and that is where you need guidance.

As your core includes all the muscles of your abdomen, your tummy muscles are the easiest muscles for people to focus on to start learning about and "retraining" their core.

Sometimes we need to give you clues as to how to use your tummy muscles, to guide your core motor control. This involves *gently* switching on your deep abdominals. That is, pulling your belly button in *a little* towards your spine. It can sometimes help to imagine that you are trying to zip up the fly on a tight pair of jeans. You need to draw your belly in so that you can pull up your zip – just don't suck in too hard, or hold your breath! *You should do this without changing your lower back position, that is without arching or flattening the back.* Most importantly you should *maintain a natural, comfortable breathing pattern.* The muscles then relax at the end of the movement pattern.

The *roller* is a great tool here as its inherent instability helps you to become aware of your abdominal muscles.

The simplest exercise you can do is to lay on your roller in the basic set up position (page 41) and breathe into your diaphragm. Slowly, quietly. Notice where your lower back is; where your neck and shoulders lie. Move your knees a little, one at a time out to the sides, and see what happens in your torso. Move your arms out to the sides, together and one at a time. Again observe what is happening in your torso. Your core will more than likely be working to stop you from falling off.

I suggest you then start some of the beginner exercises, such as the bent knee fallout and single knee lift, to further enhance your understanding of your core.

The Physio on a Roll website also has a video demonstrating core activation.

CHAPTER 3

Ready to Roll – the "how to" guide

The exercises in this book focus on stability, strength and mobility. They blend fitness-type moves with strength and Pilates-type exercises. Most are exercises that have stood the test of time, such as squats, lunges, hinges, lifts, pushes, pulls, twists and carries. These movements are actually the most useful for us as humans to perform and perfect, as they simulate the actions that we do in everyday life. Exercises that help us to move better in our day-to-day life and improve our strength, endurance or tolerance are considered functional exercises.

Generally, whenever you start a new exercise regime, it is wise to start slowly and with the basics or beginner exercises. This is especially the case if you are returning to exercise after a back, neck or joint issue or are exercising with chronic pain. Master the basics before attempting the intermediate or advanced exercises. Think of the KISS principle (Keep It Simple Stupid!). Build your capacity and control first and add complexity later.

How to use this book

This book has six exercise sections. The first four sections, Chapters 4-7 describe in detail all the exercises in the book, organised by the degree of difficulty. It is important to *choose the right movement level.*

- **Roller rookies =** beginner exercisers – you may be experiencing pain or returning to exercise after recovering from pain/injury. You may be new to exercising with a roller. The exercises in this chapter have very detailed explanations, many give specific cues about your deep tummy contractions and breathing. These exercises are gentle enough to do every day or every second day.

- **On a roll =** intermediate level. You have minimal or no pain with an average level of fitness. Aim for 2-3 sessions/week.

- **High rollers =** advanced exercisers. You have no pain and are a regular exerciser with a good fitness level. You are looking to add some complexity to your routine by introducing a roller. Up to 3 sessions/week would help with strength gains. It is important to have a rest day in between, especially if you are lifting weights. NB. You could also use your roller to stretch and massage your sore muscles.

- **Roll and release =** mobility exercises. These exercises are suitable for any level of experience and can also be performed pre- or post- any exercise session. You can do daily sessions if you desire.

Each exercise featured in these four sections has a photo (or several photos) and a description, set up, steps, tips and options for making it harder/easier.

The fifth exercise section, Chapter 8, contains:

6 specific workouts - with suggested exercises to tackle common complaints:

- **Banish your back pain** – ideal for addressing low back pain, improving abdominal and glute strength and spinal mobility.
- **No more neck pain** – helps to build deep neck strength and "switch off" unwanted muscle tension.
- **Lower limb legend** – improve your quad, core and glute strength.
- **Ultimate upper body** – targets strength in your shoulders, deep neck and core.
- **Turbo charge your core –** a great workout for your entire body.
- **Boost your balance** – how steady are you?

Chapter 9 has the sixth exercise section with **3 graded exercise programs:**

- **Benefit from the basics –** a straightforward roller workout that focuses on basic roller exercises.
- **Anything but average –** an intermediate routine that will suit those of reasonable fitness with minimal pain.
- **Roller challenge –** a workout that requires a good level of fitness that will provide a total body workout and challenge your core.

Chapters 8 and 9 will list the exercises with recommended sets and reps and a page reference. You should refer back to the relevant exercise in the previous chapters for a full description. A glossary at the rear of the book also explains terms that you may not be familiar with.

Remember: Don't fit your body to the exercise, fit the exercise to your body. Use the exercises that allow you to work the hardest with the least discomfort during and after training.

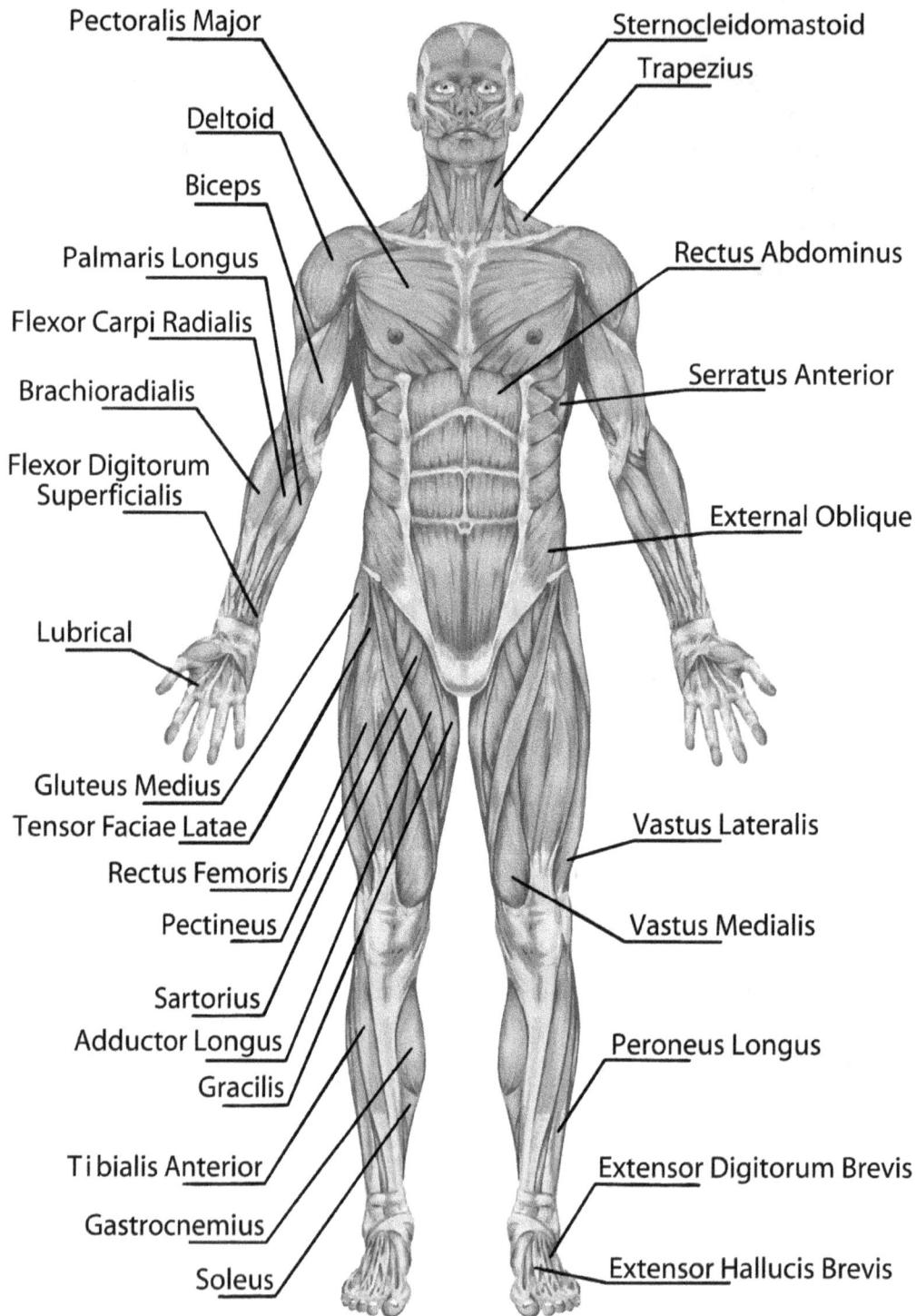

Pectoralis Major

Deltoid

Biceps

Palmaris Longus

Flexor Carpi Radialis

Brachioradialis

Flexor Digitorum
Superficialis

Lubrical

Gluteus Medius

Tensor Faciae Latae

Rectus Femoris

Pectineus

Sartorius

Adductor Longus

Gracilis

Ti bialis Anterior

Gastrocnemius

Soleus

Sternocleidomastoid

Trapezius

Rectus Abdominus

Serratus Anterior

External Oblique

Vastus Lateralis

Vastus Medialis

Peroneus Longus

Extensor Digitorum Brevis

Extensor Hallucis Brevis

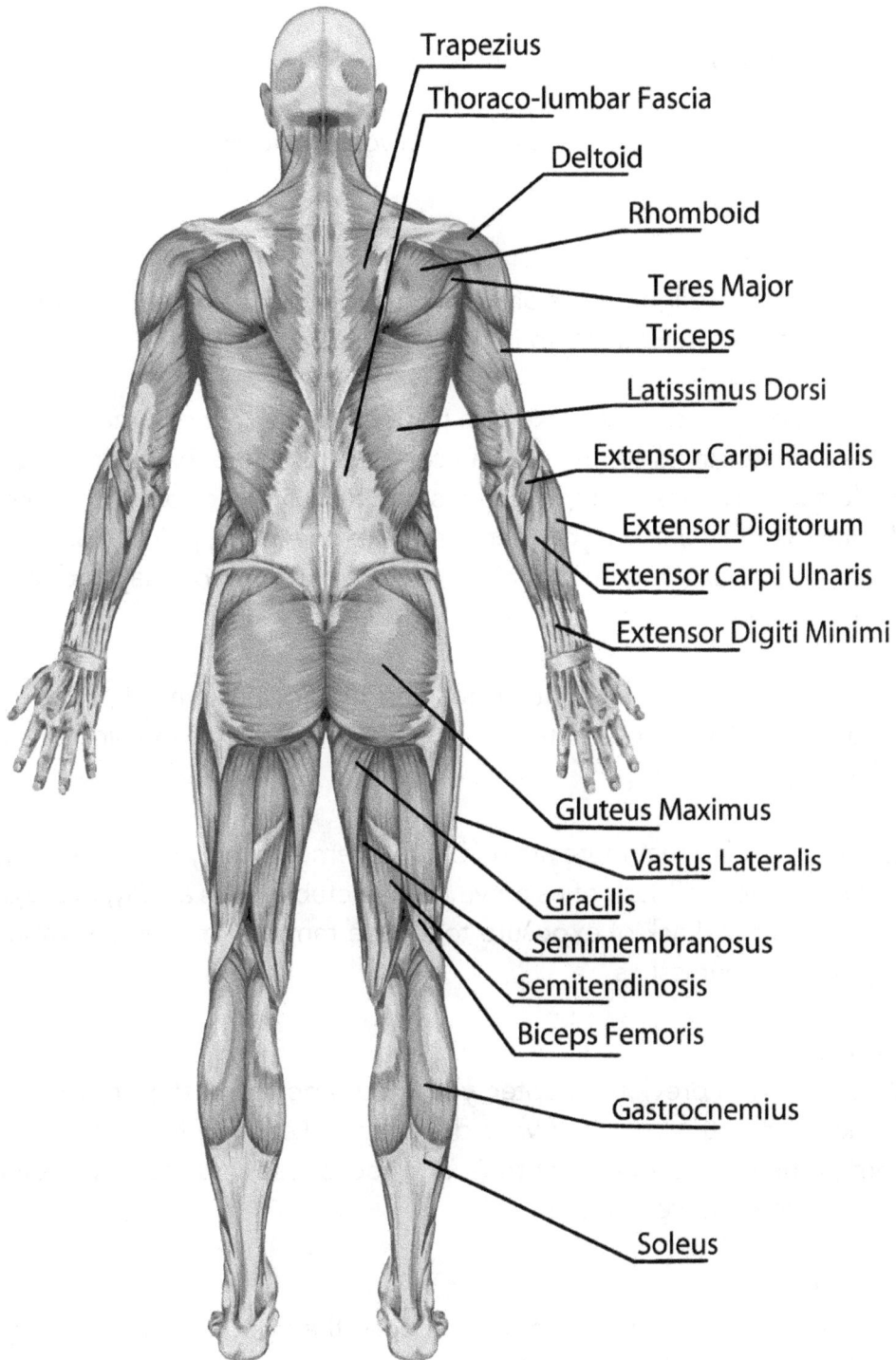

Trapezius

Thoraco-lumbar Fascia

Deltoid

Rhomboid

Teres Major

Triceps

Latissimus Dorsi

Extensor Carpi Radialis

Extensor Digitorum

Extensor Carpi Ulnaris

Extensor Digiti Minimi

Gluteus Maximus

Vastus Lateralis

Gracilis

Semimembranosus

Semitendinosis

Biceps Femoris

Gastrocnemius

Soleus

Setting up for success

To get the most out of your exercise session you should read through the following tips.

Alignment

The importance of alignment is obvious on paper, but it sometimes goes out the window once you are caught up in the exercise.

Nobody is going to do every exercise perfectly. In fact, the human body is very adept at compensating so that you can continue to do the things that you want to do. Unfortunately, those compensations don't always lead to the best outcomes or efficient biomechanics. If you then try to exercise (push, pull or twist) with poor biomechanics and/or dysfunctional movement patterns you may end up with an ache or a twinge.

The exercises in *Let it Roll* contain detailed tips for ensuring that you position your body well. This is to ensure you have the best chance of using the desired muscles.

Please keep in mind that there are no bad movements, only movements that you are not prepared for. Many of us move in predictable ways all day, every day and when we exercise. Lack of exposure to a wide range of movement variations is what can cause our issues.

Breathing

As detailed in the previous chapter, you should be trying to perform a smooth and efficient breath down into your diaphragm. Learning to breathe with your movement helps you to concentrate and focus, use your core and ultimately leads to a better movement.

Equipment

- Weights – 2/3 sets (see how to choose the right sized weight page 37)
- 90cm long x 15cm diameter roller (see foam roller basics, page 39)

- Variety of resistance bands (heavy resistance for stretches, light resistance if you have neck pain, medium resistance for strengthening)
- Small soft ball (diameter around 10cm)
- Yoga mat
- Pillow

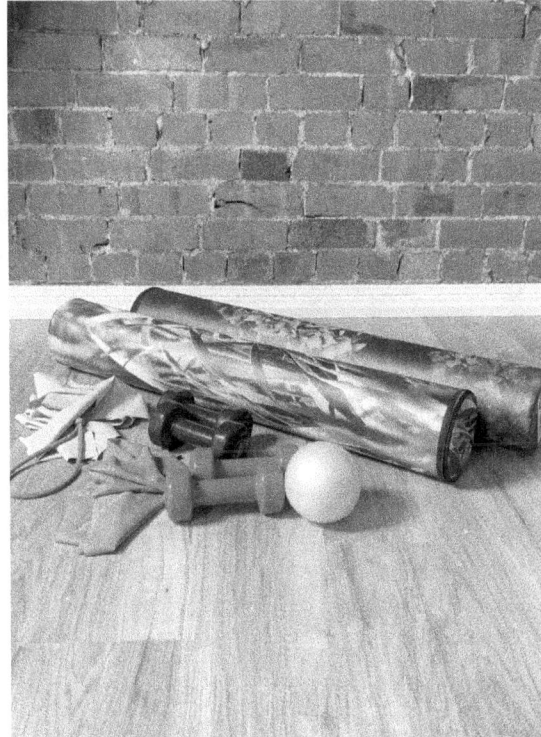

Read through the exercise

Make sure you understand what you will be doing, the alignment tips, what equipment you will need and the number of reps required. Each exercise will have suggestions for making it easier or harder.

Reps and sets

A repetition is a single performance of an exercise, e.g. one squat is a single repetition.

A set is a series of repetitions. If you do 3 sets of 8 reps of squats (3x8) you are doing 8 squats, with a rest in-between of around 30-60 seconds, then another set of 8 squats, then a rest, then another set of 8 squats.

Choose the right size weight

You should look at the recommended rep range and be able to lift your weights accordingly.

Ideally you should use a weight that you can comfortably lift 8-10x before your muscles get tired. If you can barely lift the weight 8x then it is too heavy. If you can lift it more than 15x then it is perhaps too light and you would need to perform more repetitions to achieve any strength gains.

Having said this it is perfectly acceptable to start a little lighter when you are a beginner and learning a new exercise so that you develop better form and confidence and minimise the chance of switching on too many muscle groups.

Similarly, it is easier to increase your weight size when you are in a supported lying position on the roller. Many of my clients with neck pain find that they can use a slightly heavier weight to do triceps on a roller than the weight they use when squatting and performing a bicep curl with a roller.

Surface

You will need to perform your workout on a hard, flat, non-slip surface. The floor is ideal. *Do not perform your roller exercises on your bed.* A yoga or Pilates mat may help to stop your feet slipping. A mat can also assist in decreasing the instability of the roller for a beginner exerciser.

Feel free to use a pillow underneath your head and neck for support when lying on a roller. This will be necessary if you have a forward head type posture and find it difficult or uncomfortable to tuck your chin slightly when lying supine on the roller.

A clear wall, at least a metre wide, is also useful for placing your roller on to do various bodyweight exercises.

Dress appropriately

You will need to wear comfortable, form-fitting clothes that will not get tangled while you are moving. You need to be able to *move your body freely* and be able to *feel your body* on the roller.

Wearing shoes or exercising in bare feet is generally up to your own personal preference. Bare feet will allow you to feel the floor during your workout. It can add to the stability required and enhance your proprioception. Wearing sports shoes during your workout is recommended if you usually wear orthotics. Similarly, wear shoes if you have foot/ankle or knee issues or are completing one of the more advanced workouts with weights. You will find a mix of exercises in this book photographed with and without sports shoes on feet.

Foam roller basics

Roller: size and shape

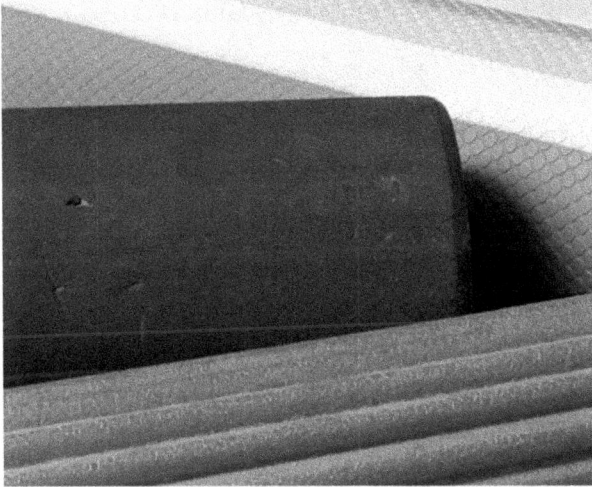

Your typical foam roller is cylindrical in shape and is made from stabilised, heat-moulded foam. It can come in a variety of different lengths, densities and diameters (and colours).

PE (polyethylene) foam rollers: these are typically the softest type of roller, are generally of lower quality and as they are not very firm, tend to distort after a short time.

EPP (expanded polypropylene) foam rollers: this is a new foam roller material on the market which looks like it is made from tightly moulded polystyrene balls with a smooth outer surface. These rollers are firm and designed for moderate to heavy use.

EVA (ethylene vinyl acetate) foam rollers: this is an excellent shock-absorbent material, very lightweight, long-lasting and hard-wearing. These rollers are ideal for continued and long- term use. An EVA foam roller will still have a slightly "spongey" feel which is ideal for people who do not want a firm foam roller. For those who require just that little bit more firmness there are high density EVA rollers which have decreased "sponginess" to create a firmer roller.

My preferred roller has a 15cm wide diameter and length of 90cm and is made from EVA foam with a hardness score of 35+. It is pictured throughout this book and is available to purchase from **Physio on a Roll.** This **Physio on a Roll** foam roller is very hard. The more dense or harder the roller the more likely it is to maintain its shape. It is also more "unstable" and as such a great core facilitator. However, if you are sensitive to pressure you should use a less dense or softer roller, then progress to a firmer roller as you are able. Another option is to use a folded towel along the length of the roller until your body gets used to the hardness. Please note that your body does adapt surprisingly quickly to the feel of a roller.

If you are still a little apprehensive about being on the roller you could use a half or hemispherical roller first.

Textured Rollers: Rollers also now come with textured external features such as waves, grids, blades, ridges and knobs. These types of rollers are almost exclusively used for stretching and myofascial releases. You could purchase a textured roller in addition to your basic roller if desired.

Similarly, short rollers (30-50cm in length) are a great idea for travel. They do fit easily into suitcases and are great for limb massage. These rollers are, however, limited in their ability to be used for most core and strengthening exercises due to their smaller length.

Vibrating rollers: these are a relatively recent addition to the roller range. They are usually battery-operated and exclusively used for massaging muscles pre- and post-exercise.

Care of the roller

Your foam roller should be stored flat to avoid it becoming warped. It should also be away from direct sunlight as UV rays can deteriorate the foam.

*Tip: behind the door or under your bed is an ideal place to store your roller (but don't forget to use your roller as out of sight should not mean out of mind!). Unless, of course, you have a **Physio on a Roll** foam roller. These are designed to be attractive enough to leave in your living/dining/lounge room where you will see it and remember to use it!*

Continuous pressure can cause dents so avoid stacking anything heavy on the roller. Clean your roller using a damp cloth. Don't use bleach, oils or any chemicals or you will damage the foam. If you have a covered roller, however, you can use sprays and antibacterial wipes to clean without fear of damage.

Basic set up lying on a roller

When beginning any exercise lying on the roller it is a great idea initially, to go through this basic set up. This will ensure that you know where your body is and that you have a greater chance of performing your exercise successfully. It is also a great beginner warm up routine.

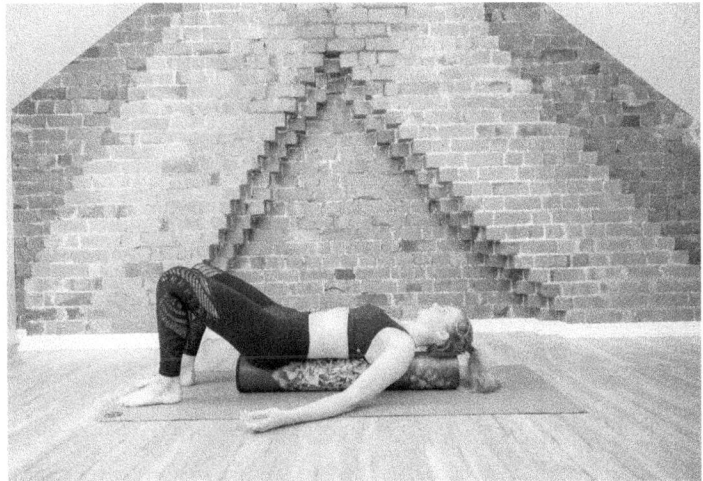

Basic set up on the foam roller as illustrated above:

- Lay on top of the roller, on your back with your bottom at one end and your head at the other.

- Your feet and knees should be hip-width apart, with your ankles more or less vertically in line with your knees.

- Your lumbar spine should be in a neutral position. To find your neutral position, pelvic tilt to touch or gently squash your lower back onto the roller. Then pelvic tilt to arch your lower back away from the roller (keeping your tailbone in contact). Keep pelvic tilting until you find the midway position. This is your "neutral" lower back or lumbar spine position. It should feel comfortable and you should be pain free.

- Place one hand on your stomach (over your belly button) and the other hand just below your sternum. Elbows can rest on the floor. You should be breathing down into your diaphragm so that you are aware of your belly gently rising and falling with your breath. Your ribs should not poke up.

- Gently tuck your chin a little to elongate your neck.

- Place both arms in the air, in line with your shoulders, palms facing each other. Reach for the ceiling, then squeeze your shoulder blades gently around the roller. Repeat this several times to relax your neck and find a neutral position where your shoulder blade muscles are very slightly engaged (around 10%). Allow your arms to then relax on the floor beside you, palms facing down.

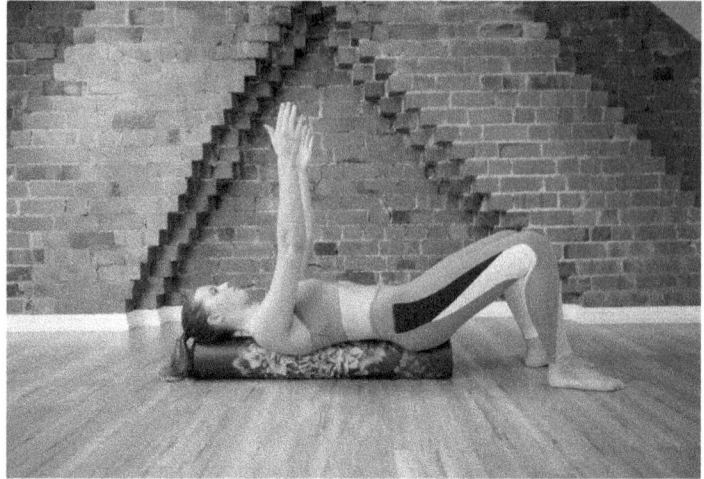

- Try to engage your deep abdominal (or tummy) muscles, at a low level, by gently drawing your belly button in, towards your spine, without moving from your neutral back position *when you breathe out.* It can sometimes help to imagine that you are trying to zip up the fly on a tight pair of jeans. You need to draw your belly in a little so that you can pull up your zip – just don't suck in too hard or hold your breath! Squeeze your tummy muscles at about 25% or less of a full contraction without pelvic tilting or turning on your surface or superficial abdominal muscles. Relax as you breathe in.

- NB. Your ribs should not flare or poke out if you are breathing normally with length in your neck and thoracic spine.

Warm up

The purpose of a warm up is to prepare your body for the exercises that are to come, increasing your body and breath awareness and gently raising your body temperature, heart rate and oxygen consumption.

The following warm up includes range of motion exercises to help mobilise your joints, neck and spine, and movement preparation exercises to activate your muscles and the nervous system before you begin your workout.

It is purposely simple for beginners and those who may have pain. A more complex warm up routine is available on the Physio on a Roll website.

You can use the same protocol before each workout and you could also add in some of the massages in the "Roll and Release" chapter before you work out. A video of the following simple warm up sequence can also be viewed on the Physio on a Roll website.

Feel free to do more on one side than the other, especially if that is where you have an issue. Most of us have discrepancies on one side or another.

STANDING

1. *Alignment awareness*
   Head over shoulders, relaxing neck and shoulders, finding your neutral lumbar spine, soften knees (not locked or hyperextended), body weight evenly distributed between heels and toes.

2. *Breathing awareness*
   Relaxed diaphragmatic breathing, through the nose, maintaining a relaxed neck and shoulders.

3. Tilt the chin to the chest, then the ear to right shoulder.

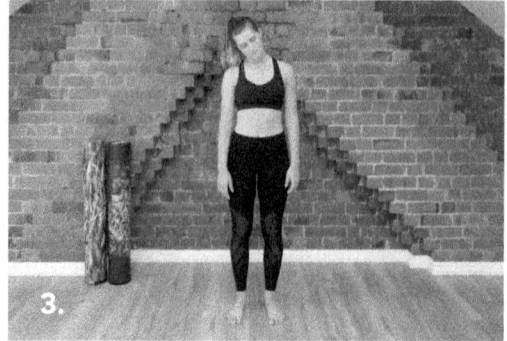

4. Stretch from the left (opposite) shoulder to the left fingertips, turning the left palm to the floor.

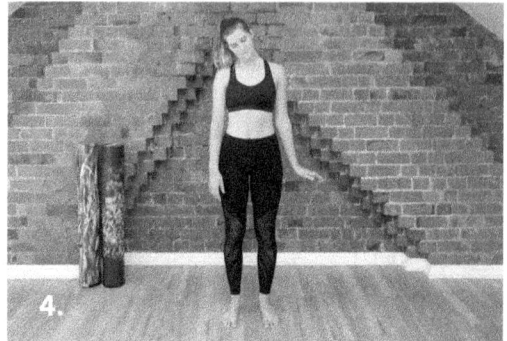

5. Maintain position 4 as you rotate the chin to armpit on the right side.

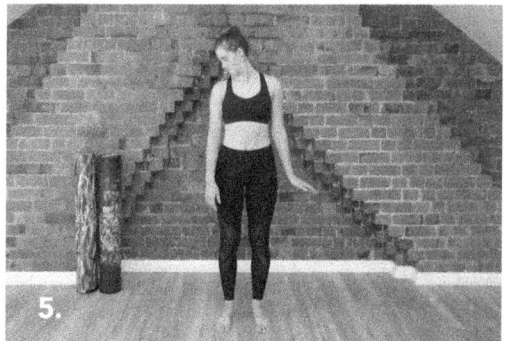

6. Repeat 3-5 with the ear tilting to the left shoulder.

7. Breathe in, link your hands, raise the hands in front of the body until they are overhead.

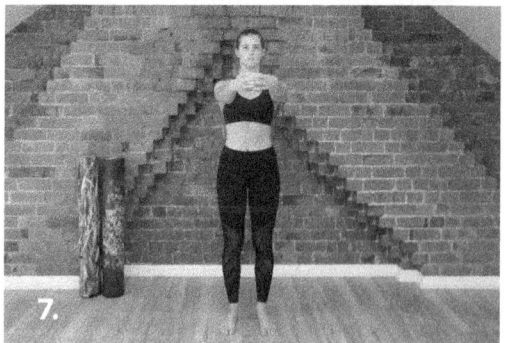

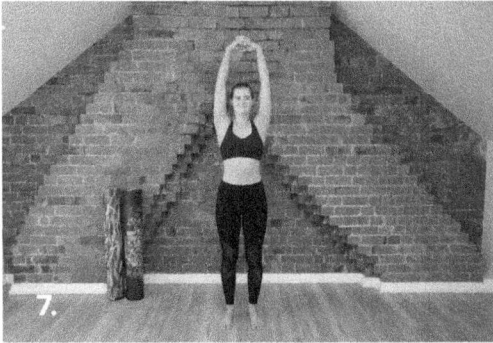

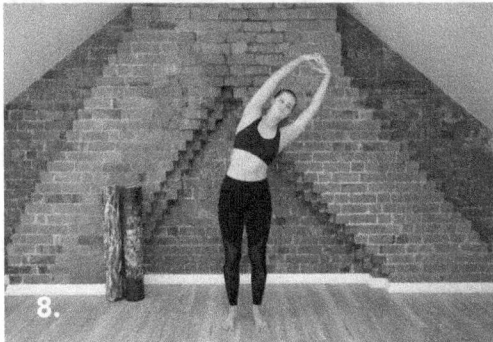

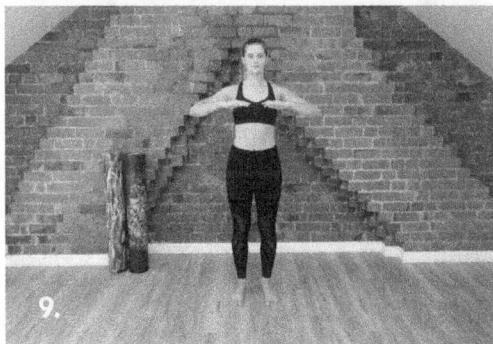

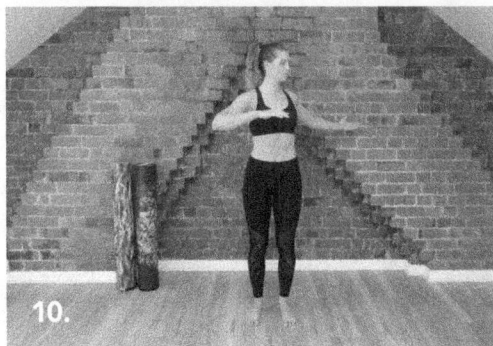

8. Breathe out as you tilt to the right, in the range that is comfortable then breathe in as you return and breathe out again as you tilt to the left, breathing in as you return. Repeat x2.

9. Lift your arms, palms down out in front of your body. Keep your hands below shoulder height, with elbows bent, gently drawing your shoulder blades down and back.

10. Breathe in and as you breathe out sweep your right arm out to the side, rotating the palm upwards as your elbow straightens. Rotate your torso but keep your hips facing forward. Your head should follow your hands. Return and repeat on the left. Repeat x2.

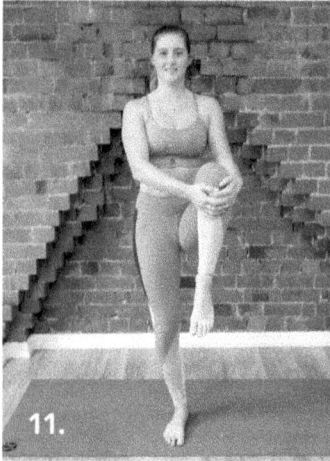

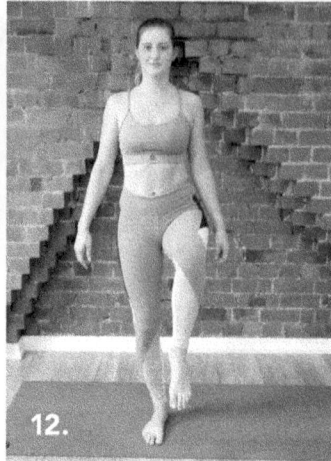

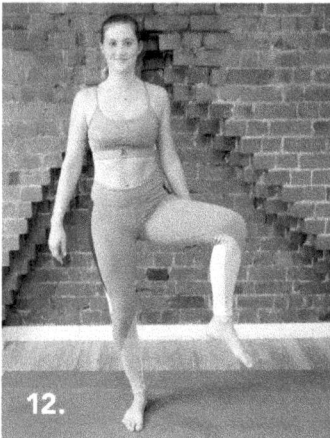

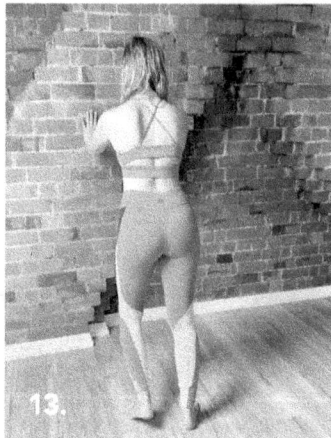

11. Keeping your right knee slightly flexed and weight into the right heel, lift your left hip and hug towards your chest. Repeat with your right hip. Repeat x2.

12. Lift your left knee to hip height, rotate out to the side, back to the centre then lower back down to the floor. Repeat x2. Repeat with the right knee (use a roller for balance if necessary).

13. Turn to face a wall, place both hands on the wall, directly in front of shoulders. Lean into the wall and draw your shoulder blades down and back and maintain as you raise and lower alternating heels x10.

Let it Roll

CHAPTER 4

Roller Rookies

"The beginning is the most important part of the work."
Plato

The following exercises are a great introduction to using the foam roller. All the exercises are straightforward, designed to make you aware of your core muscles and how they work together to stabilise your body and help you move. It may be worthwhile to re-read "basic core activation" if you are at all unsure which muscles you will be using and why.

You can do more or less than the recommended reps. If you find any of the basic roller exercises difficult or painful, try the exercise without the roller, then re-introduce the roller. There should be no back or neck pain or discomfort while performing each exercise. Bridging and the neck exercises don't include a roller as you will achieve more at a beginner level, roller free.

Remember to read through the exercise fully before commencing so that you know what compensations to look out for. It is also worth remembering that each exercise has a video that can be viewed online via the Physio on a Roll website.

BENT KNEE FALL OUT

Bent knee fall out is the simplest abdominal exercise you can do on the roller. It is perfect for beginners, as you learn about how your deep abdominal muscles work.

Set up:

- Supine on the roller, head resting at one end, bottom at the other.
- Feet and knees hip-width apart, lumbar spine neutral.
- Practise, as you breathe out, drawing your belly button in towards spine at about 25% of a contraction, without changing your lower back position.
- Gently tuck your chin and have your shoulder blade muscles slightly contracted.
- Forearms resting lightly on the floor.
- Breathe normally down into your diaphragm.

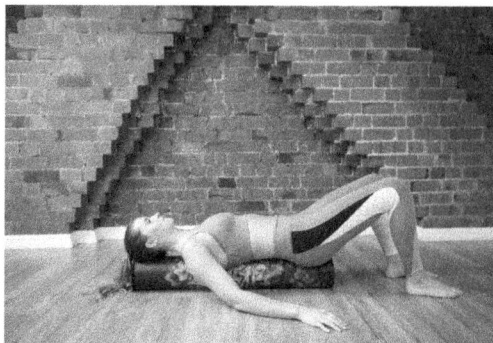

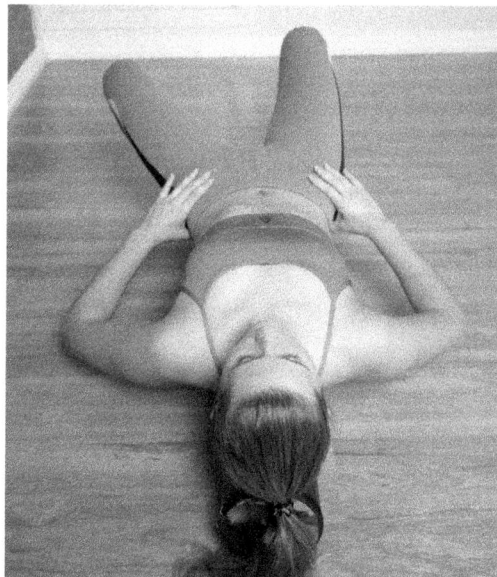

Steps:

1. Breathe in and as you breathe out slowly move your right knee out to the right side (somewhere between 1 and 2 o'clock if you think of a clock analogy) and then breathe in and return to your starting position.
2. Breathe out and move the left knee out to somewhere between

10 and 11 o'clock and then breathe in as you return to your starting position.

3. Repeat 10 times (x10) each side, alternating sides.
4. Do 2-3 sets with a 30-second rest in between sets.

Tips:

- Tummy contraction should remain at a low 25% or less of a contraction throughout the exercise – you should not feel that you are using your upper abdominal muscles.
- There should be no rocking or rotation of your pelvis or loss of your neutral back position, i.e. don't actively squash your back into the roller or arch your lower back away from the roller.
- Remember to breathe normally throughout so that upper abdominal muscles remain relaxed, with no rib flaring. If you breathe differently to the instructions above that is okay, just don't hold your breath!
- Keep your neck and shoulders relaxed.

Make it harder:
- Progress to only elbow support on the floor, repeat as above.
- Progress to no arms on the floor, hands resting lightly on stomach, repeat as above.
- Perform bent knee fall out with a resistance band around the tops of the knees, repeat as above.

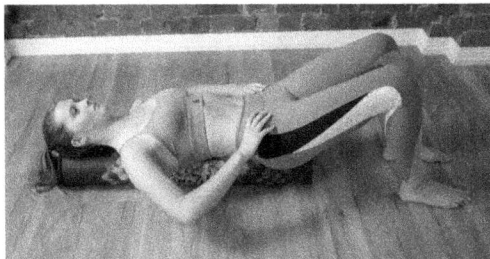

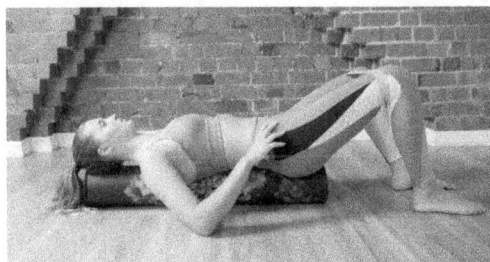

SINGLE KNEE LIFT

Single knee lift is the second basic abdominal exercise that suits beginner to intermediate exercisers on the roller. Make this exercise easier or harder by changing the amount of arm support you use on the floor.

Set up:
- Supine on roller, with feet and knees hip-width apart.
- Neutral lumbar spine.
- Chin tucked a little, shoulder blade muscles slightly contracted.
- Forearms resting lightly on the floor.

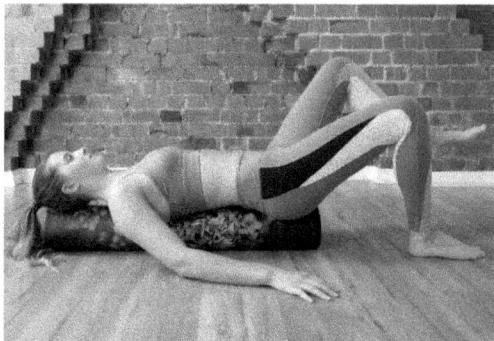

Steps:
1. Breathe in, then as you breathe out slowly lift the right knee above the right hip.
2. Then breathe in and slowly lower the foot back to the floor.
3. Then breathe out and slowly and gently lift the left knee above the left hip, then breathe in and lower the foot slowly back to the floor.
4. Continue to alternate the knee lifts.
5. Repeat x10 each side. 2-3 sets.

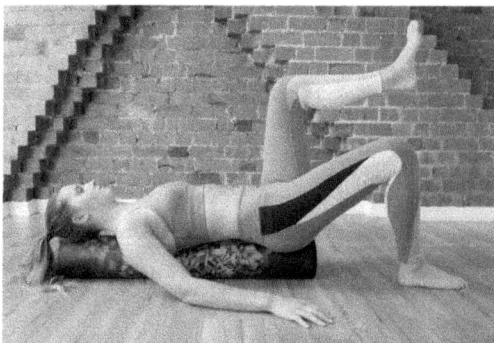

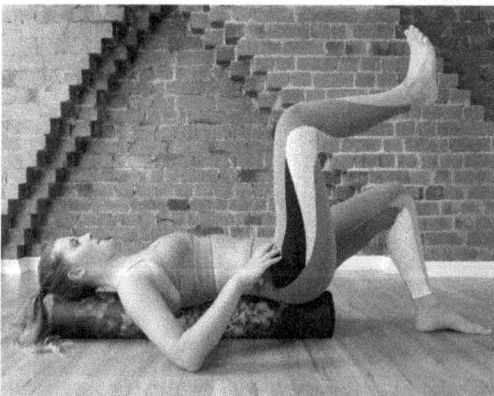

Tips:
- Take care to place the foot on the floor directly in front of the same hip so that the feet don't get closer and closer together and create a smaller base of support.

- You can maintain your low-level deep tummy contraction throughout the exercise; *you may be already starting to do this automatically with your breathing.* This will help keep your lower back in a neutral position throughout, i.e. your lumbar spine shouldn't lift or lower on the roller, especially as you swap legs.
- Make sure you breathe with each movement, i.e. lift the leg as you breathe out, breathe in as you lower.
- Don't allow any excess movement through your trunk or pelvis or let your tummy "blow out" or ribs pop, especially as you swap legs.
- Keep neck and shoulders relaxed throughout.
- There should be no back pain.

Make it harder:
- Progress to elbow support only on the floor
- Then try no arm support on floor, with hands resting lightly on stomach.

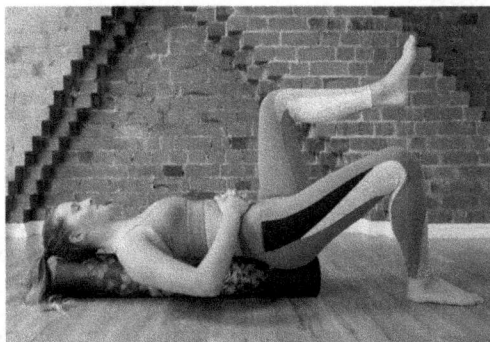

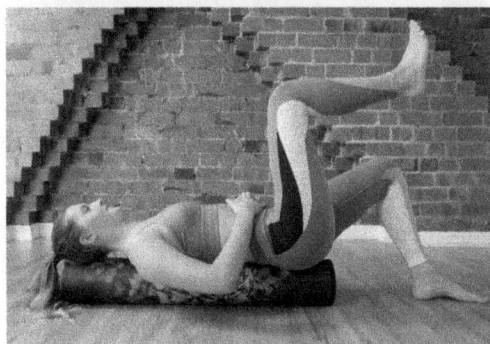

SINGLE LEG EXTENSION

Single leg extension on the roller is a simple progression of the single knee lift exercise. By extending (straightening) your knee, a longer lever is created, requiring more core control.

Set up:
- Supine on the roller, feet and knees hip-width apart.
- Neutral lumbar spine.
- Chin tucked a little, shoulder blade muscles slightly contracted.
- Forearms resting lightly on the floor.

Steps:
1. Breathe in and then as you breathe out lift the right knee over the right hip.
2. Breathe in and straighten the right knee.
3. Breathe out as you slowly lower your leg towards the floor. You should stop when your leg is parallel to the floor; try not to touch the floor.
4. Breathe in and bend the knee and bring it back over the right hip.
5. Then as you breathe out, lower the right foot back to the floor.
6. Breathe in and as you breathe out lift the left knee over the left hip.
7. Continue as above.
8. Repeat x10-20, alternating legs. 2 sets.

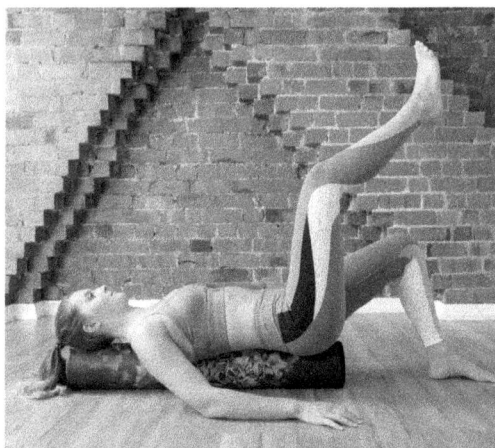

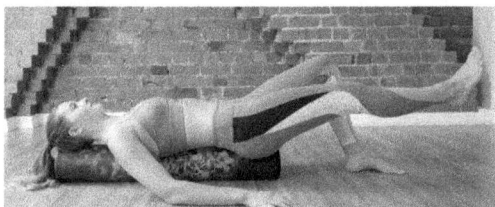

Tips:

- Try to lower the foot to the floor directly in front of the corresponding hip. This will help you to maintain your hip-width distance between your feet and help with your stability.
- Try to keep your lower back in a neutral position, so that it does not arch or flatten on the roller. This is especially important as you swap from one leg to the other, when you will feel most unsteady.
- Continue to breathe normally throughout the exercise. Don't worry too much about when to breathe at this stage – if that is too hard, just remember to breathe consistently.
- Try not to let your ribs "pop".
- Keep your neck and shoulders relaxed throughout the exercise; there should be no neck or back pain. If there is, go back to single knee lift and practice more repetitions.

Make it harder:

- Progress to elbow support only on the floor.
- Try no arm support on the floor, with hands resting lightly on your stomach.
- Repeat on the same leg x10, then the other leg x10.
- Progress to an intermediate exercise of dead bug abdominals on the roller.

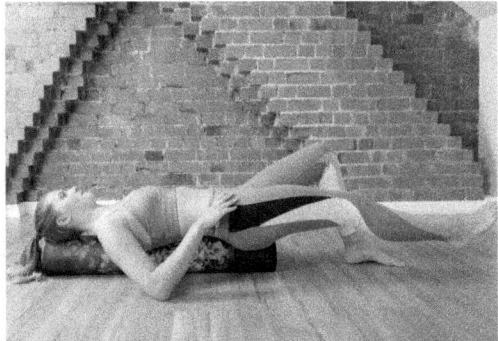

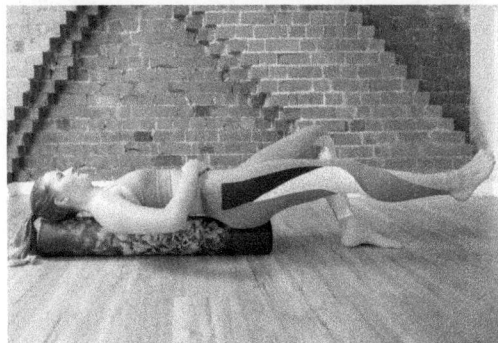

ROLLER ABDOMINALS – HANDS OVERHEAD (VARIATIONS)

Another abdominal exercise this time using the roller in your hands. Progress easily from a beginner exercise right through to an advanced abdominal workout by changing your leg positions.

Set up:
- Supine lying on a flat surface, with knees bent, feet and knees hip-width apart.
- Neutral lumbar spine.
- Chin slightly tucked and neck lengthened, head on or off a pillow as desired.
- Hands on each end of the roller, with the roller resting horizontally on the tummy.

Steps:
1. Raise the roller over your chest so that your hands on the ends of the roller are in line with your shoulders.
2. Gently contract your deep tummy, keeping ribs flat, as you breathe out and slowly lower the roller behind your head, touching the floor lightly.
3. Then return to hands over your chest while breathing in.
4. Repeat x10, with each repetition now stopping just short of touching the floor.
5. Repeat 2-3 sets, resting the roller lightly on your tummy between sets.

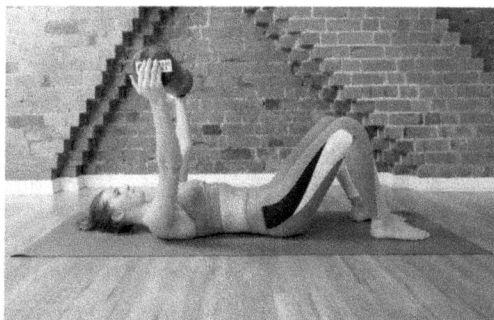

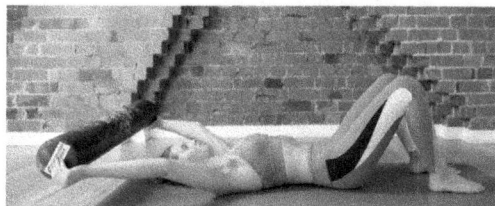

Let it Roll

Tips:

- Make sure that you breathe into the diaphragm throughout.
- Relax your neck and shoulders, i.e. try to let your shoulders roll in their sockets, do not let them lift up towards your ears.
- Do not let your ribs "pop", i.e. the thoracic spine at mid chest should stay lengthened.
- There should be no back pain or neck pain. If you do experience pain you should check your positioning. You could also use a small pillow under the lower back for support. Alternatively, go back to a basic abdominal exercise such as single knee lift.

Make it harder:

- Raise your right knee over your right hip and hold this position as you move the roller behind your head x10 repetitions, then repeat on the left. 2-3 sets.
- Lift your right knee over your right hip and then extend/straighten your right knee towards the floor (but do not touch the floor) as the roller goes behind your head x10 repetitions. Repeat on the left. 2-3 sets.

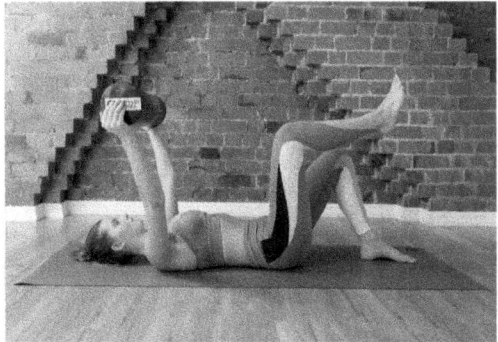

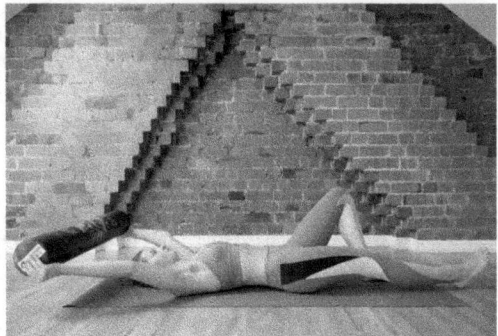

WALL PUSH-UP WITH A ROLLER

This is a great starter push-up for those with neck, shoulder or back issues. It works your core, upper body and especially your shoulders. Good shoulder strength is particularly important if you suffer from neck pain – as you will be less likely to overuse those big surface neck muscles if your upper body is strong.

Set up:
- In standing, facing a wall about an arms-length away.
- Feet parallel and feet and knees hip-width apart.
- Lumbar spine neutral, deep tummy contracted at a low level.
- Roller placed horizontally on a wall, *at shoulder height or slightly lower.*
- Both hands on the roller (with thumbs adjacent to fingers, not stretched around the roller) wider than shoulder-width apart.
- Elbows straight (i.e. extended) but not locked. *NB. If you suffer from neck pain, start with your elbows flexed.*

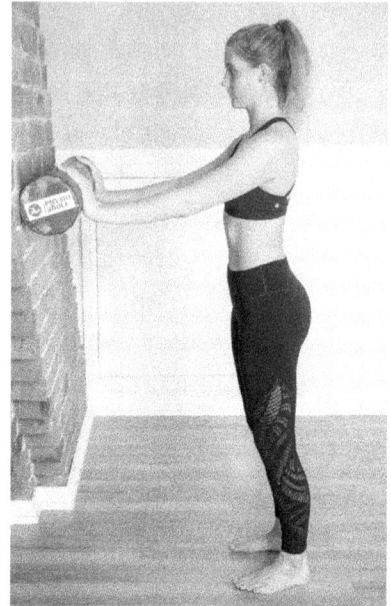

Steps:
1. Lean your body weight through your arms gently onto the roller, onto the wall, maintaining elbow extension.
2. Gently contract your shoulder blade muscles, i.e. squeeze them together, drawing them down and back a little, and maintain this slight contraction.
3. Then breathe in, bend your elbows and lower your chest towards roller, maintaining

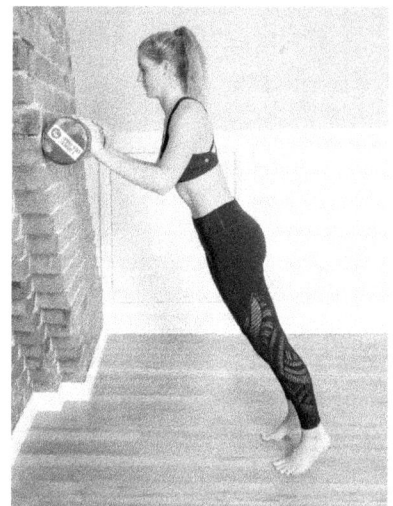

your gentle deep tummy contraction and your gentle shoulder blade contraction throughout.

4. Your head should stay in line with your body. Don't poke your chin out.
5. Breathe out, straighten your elbows and return to the starting position.
6. Repeat x10. 2-3 sets.

Tips:
- The roller is a cylindrical object on a flat wall so you need to maintain pressure on it to stop it slipping down the wall while you perform your basic push-up.
- Your upper neck muscles need to stay relaxed. If you can feel them working, bend your elbows and/or move your feet closer to the wall and/or lower the roller on the wall.
- There should be no neck or back pain, just shoulder fatigue.
- Try not to let your hips sag forward. Maintain alignment through your ear, shoulder, hips and knees and ankles.
- Do your push-up without a roller following the same instructions if you are still having difficulty.

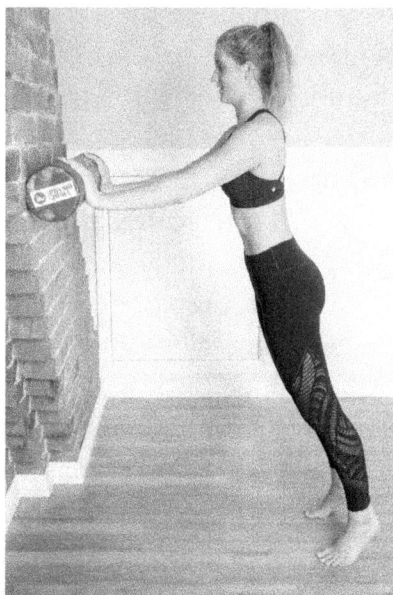

Make it harder:
- Rise up onto your toes and perform the wall push-up on a roller as described above.
- Rise up onto your toes and then extend one leg, from the hip, behind you, toes on the floor. Perform push-up as described above x10 and then repeat with other leg extended x10.

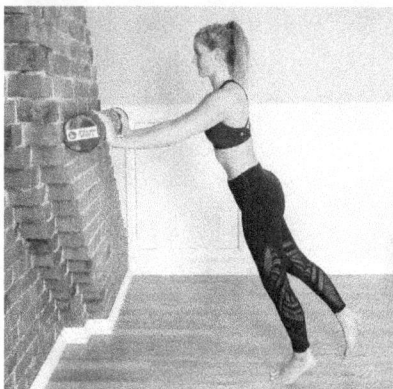

GLUTES WITH A ROLLER

This exercise is a functional gluteal strengthener. By activating your glutes in a single leg standing position, your brain is more likely to switch on your glutes in other real-life single leg scenarios (26). A great example is stepping up a staircase. You need your glutes to work consistently to keep your pelvis stable as you take each alternate step. In this way, basic glutes with a roller demonstrates a skill process I described in Chapter 3, "Before you Roll", as motor control.

NB. This glutes with a roller exercise can be quite difficult to master. It can be simplified and performed in stages (see tips). Please take your time with the set up. It is detailed but if followed correctly results in a great butt burn!

Set up
- Place your roller on the wall horizontally, at hip level, parallel with the floor.
- Stand side-on to the wall and the roller, and place your hip (about where you would put your hand in your pocket) halfway along the length of the roller.
- Look down and check that your feet are hip-width apart. Feet should also be level and your outside foot should line up with your outside hip.
- Both your knees should be slightly bent.
- Then look straight ahead. Your ears should be aligned over your shoulders, shoulders aligned over your hips.
- Shoulder blade muscles should be gently contracted and neck should be relaxed. Breathe normally.

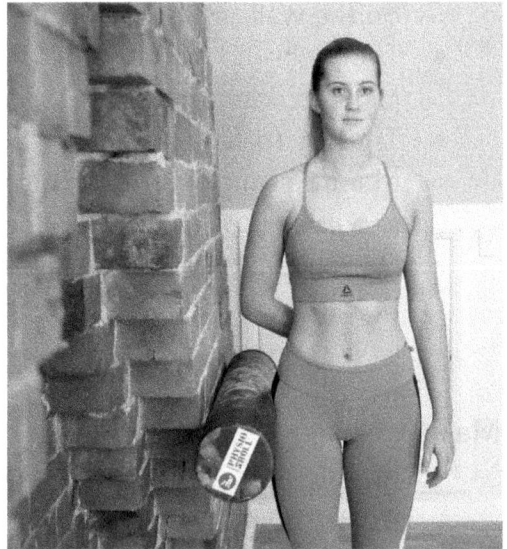

Steps:

1. Push sideways with your hips into the roller, onto the wall.
2. Maintain the sideways push into the roller as you lift your *inside heel* **only** off the floor (at this stage you should be aware of the muscles in your outside glute starting to contract).
3. Lift the *entire inside foot off the floor* (the glute contraction should feel stronger).
4. Maintain the hip pressure on the roller on the wall as you gently *roll your inside hip up the wall a little*. Hold this hitched up position, feeling the glute contraction on the outside *feeling stronger again*.
5. Hold this position to fatigue.
6. Repeat on the other side.

Tips:

- If you feel pain in the outside hip or running down the outside thigh, stop and check your body positioning and start again.
- If you are still having difficulty activating your outside buttock, stop at the stage where you do feel a contraction and hold to fatigue.
- Try to keep your body weight into your heel on the outside foot and keep a slight bend in the outside knee.
- Don't change your neutral lumbar spine. Check your lower back position

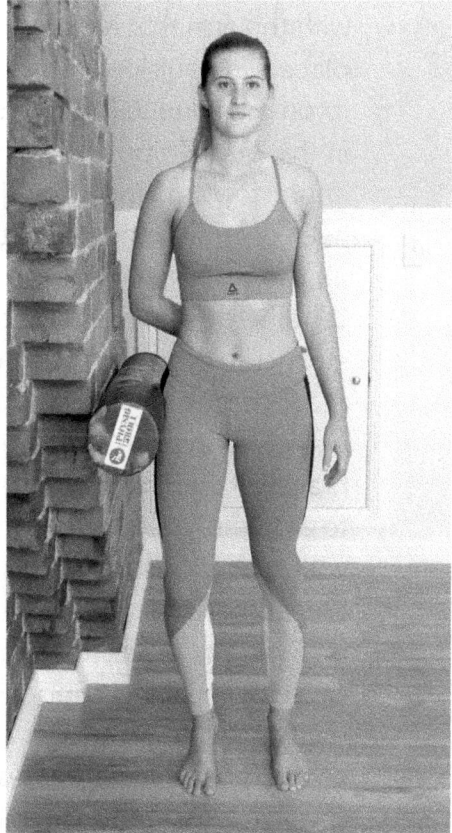

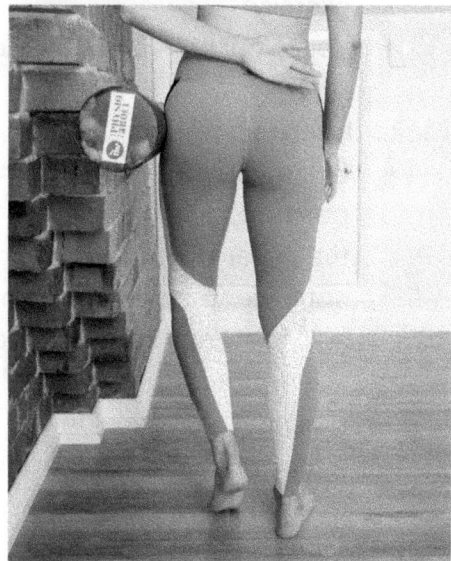

with the arm that is closest to the wall placed in your low back.

- If you continue to lose the contraction in the outside butt when you lift the entire foot off the floor, just lift the heel only and then add the hip roll up the wall and hold.

- When you have a buttock that is stronger or contracts better than the other, that buttock should be exercised on the outside first. Your brain will then have a better idea how to activate your weaker glutes when you swap sides.

- Sometimes you may find that the roller is too firm to push into or that doing so causes pain. If this happens, swap the roller for a small diameter squashy ball and follow the same process as above.

- Breathe normally throughout the exercise.

- Keep your neck and shoulders relaxed.

Make it harder:
- Once you have held the hip hitched position for 20 seconds, slowly roll the roller down the wall a little (but not lower than your starting position) and then roll back up and continue slowly until you fatigue. Maintain the sideways pressure on the hip on the roller on the wall throughout.

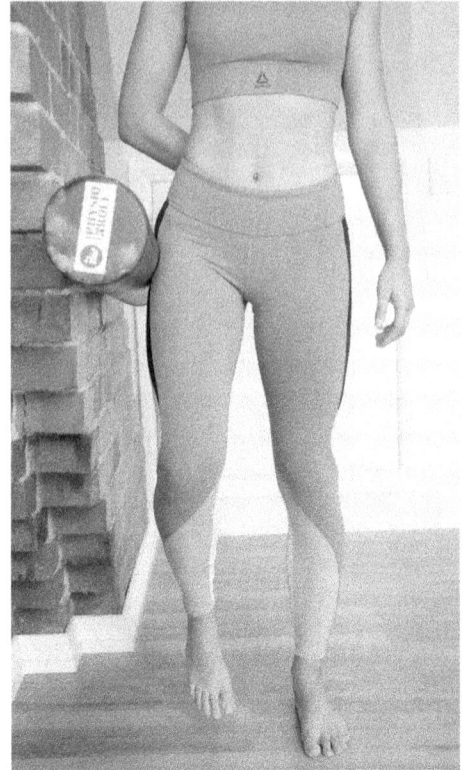

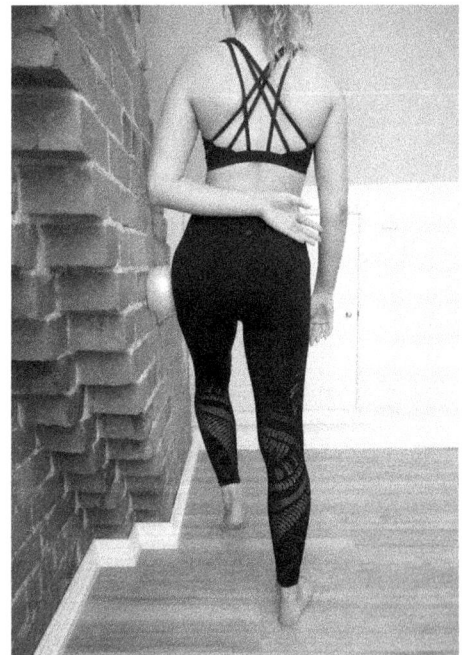

BASIC WALL SQUAT WITH A ROLLER

This wall squat is a simple and functional quads, gluteal and core strengthening exercise. The roller guides your squat, as it sits comfortably in your lumbar spine. It allows you to focus on your hip and knee flexion knowing that your lumbar spine is supported and positioned optimally. Adding hand weights adds variety and also challenges the upper torso, particularly the shoulder and core.

Set up:

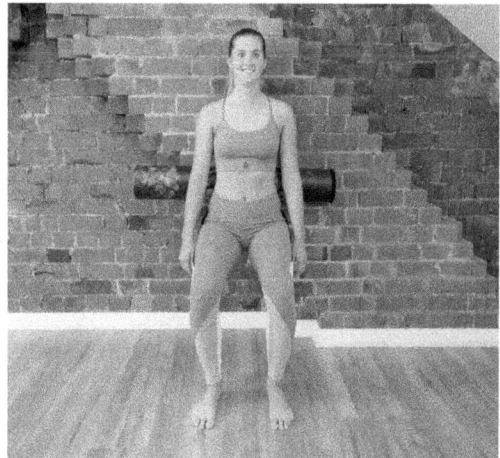

- Place your roller on a wall, horizontally.
- Place your lumbar spine area (see tips) on the roller, on the wall.
- Knees should be bent, with your feet and knees hip-width apart, and your feet further out from the wall than your knees.
- The centre of each kneecap should line up with the second toe (the toe next to the big toe) of each foot.
- Your head should be neutral, with your ears lined up over your mid-shoulder, shoulders over hips, lumbar spine neutral.
- Weights, if using, in your hands, arms beside your upper body.

Steps:

1. Breathe in and bend your knees and hips and lower your buttocks towards the floor, rolling the roller on the wall.
2. Lower *in the range that is comfortable*, but not going past knee height.
3. Breathe out and push into your heels, straighten your knees and hips and roll back up to the starting position.
4. Repeat x15-20. 2 sets.
5. You should feel mostly thighs and buttocks working.

Tips:

- Do not lean on or away from the roller; that is, your lumbar spine should stay neutral throughout and hips should stay in line with shoulders (side-on view). The roller should guide your squat.
- Don't let your knees roll out to the side or in towards each other; this can cause knee pain or clicking (use a small ball between the knees if you have difficulty maintaining your knee alignment).
- Keep weight into your heels, especially as you straighten your knees on return to your starting position.
- Keep your neck and shoulders relaxed.

Make it harder:

- Add in appropriately sized hand weights and perform any of the following with the squat – bicep curls, shoulder forward flexion to 90°, lateral raise to 90°, scaption, overhead press.
- Use the weight in one hand only, performing all the repetitions on one side only and then changing sides to challenge the core.
- Increase the repetitions up to 40 with weights as above.
- Maintain the low point of the squat

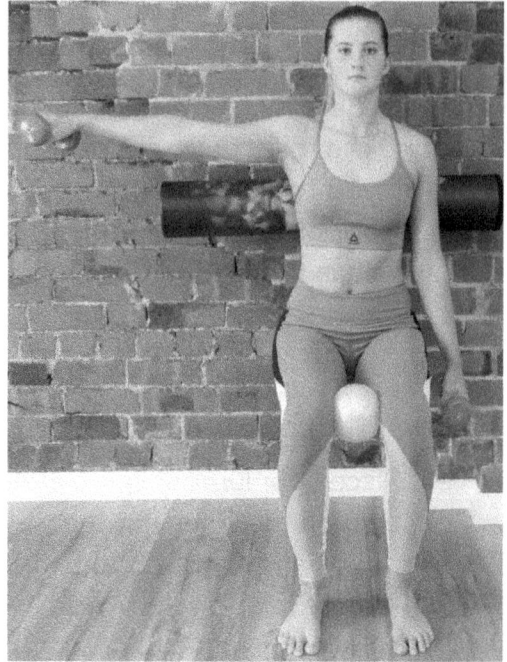

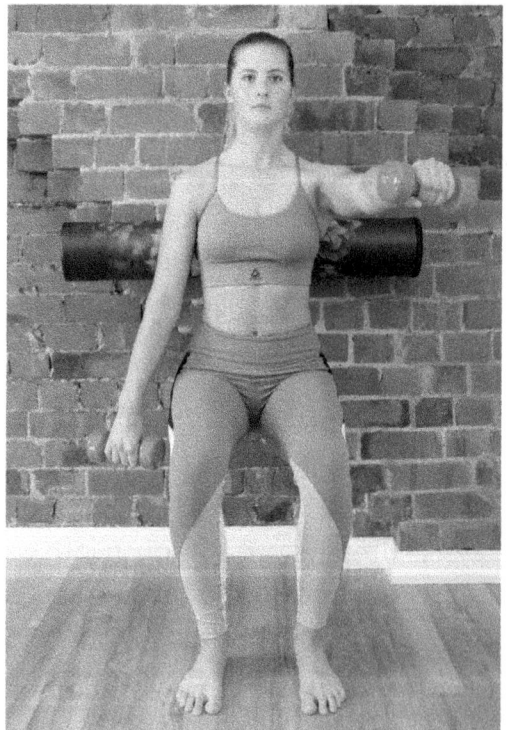

(a sustained squat) and perform any of the weighted exercises as above.

- Try a sustained wall squat (see Physio on a Roll website).
- Use a resistance band in your hands or under the balls of your feet to perform bicep curls, lateral raises, shoulder forward flexion, and scaption while squatting or holding a static squat.

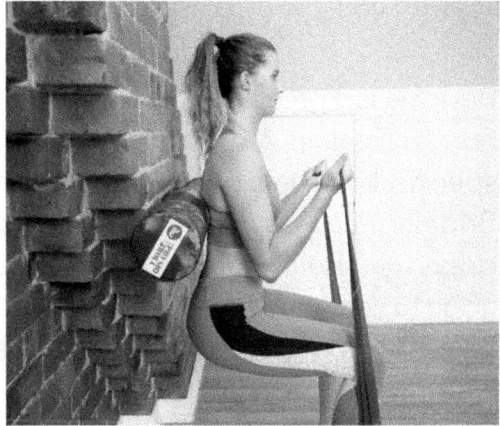

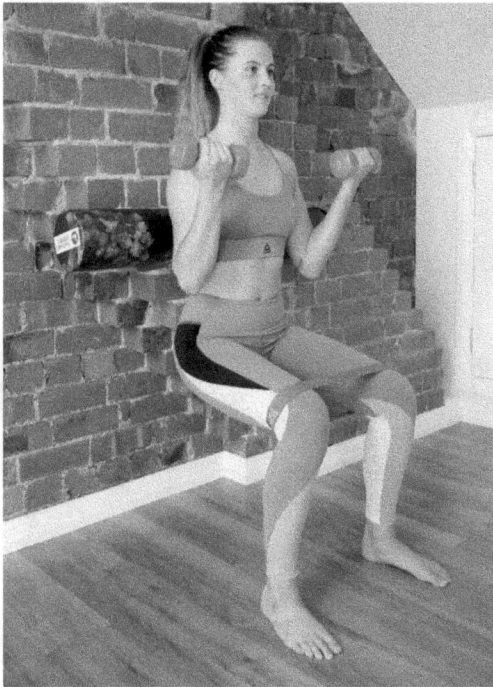

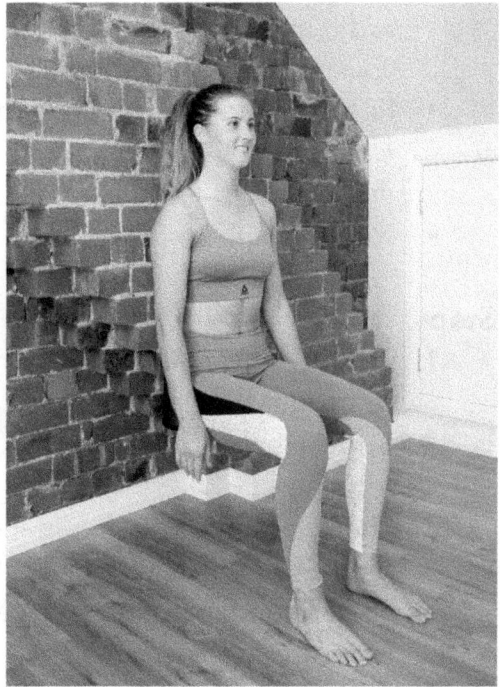

BASIC BRIDGE

Bridging is a great foundational exercise to master if you suffer from low back pain. For that reason, I have included it in the basic section without a roller initially. It specifically targets glutes and core and helps you to improve your spinal mobility. Bridging teaches you how to use your glutes and move your pelvis. It is also a great exercise if you have hip or knee soreness as improving your glute strength adds to your stability at your hip and knee. The bridge, once mastered, can then be easily progressed with or without equipment to be quite an advanced exercise.

Set up:

- In a crook lying position, supine on the floor, feet and knees hip-width apart, your arms relaxed by your sides, palms facing up.
- Feet should be drawn *slightly closer to the bottom (closer than in the photo).*
- Neutral lumbar spine.

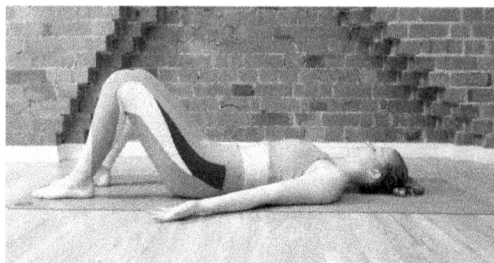

Steps:

1. *Tilt the pelvis* to flatten the lumbar spine into the floor.
2. *Squeeze the bottom* muscles together.
3. Then *push into your heels* and *lift the bottom* off the floor until the shoulders, hips and knees align (side-on view).
4. Pause, but keep squeezing the bottom muscles.
5. Then slowly lower your body down to the floor, one vertebra at a time until the tailbone touches the floor.
6. Repeat x6-8. 2-3 sets.

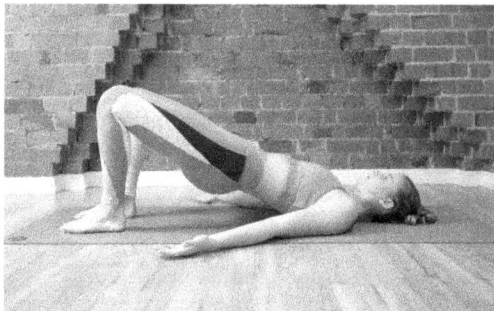

Tips:

- The hamstrings (muscles at the back of your thighs) **should not** be working hard. If they are, *move your feet closer to your bottom* (but not touching the bottom). Make sure you keep pressure into the heels throughout the bridge.
- Your lower back should not hurt. Do not lift the hips too high or you may lose your neutral back position and arch too far.
- Relax your neck and shoulders. Even though you are weight-bearing on your shoulders they should not end up near your ears.
- Don't hold your breath.

Make it harder:

- Hold the elevated position for a count of 3 before slowly descending.
- Increase the reps to x10 and do 3 sets.
- In the elevated position, do alternating heel lifts. Perform 3 on each side before returning to the floor. Do 5 sets.
- Add a resistance band around the knees (or just above or below) and once in the elevated bridge position do 3-5 unilateral or bilateral bent knee fallouts before slowly lowering back to the start. Repeat x3-5.
- Add in a roller, *basic bridge with a roller (page 95)* or at the feet *roller bridges (page 134)*.

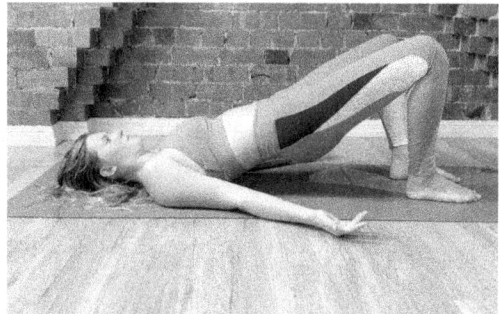

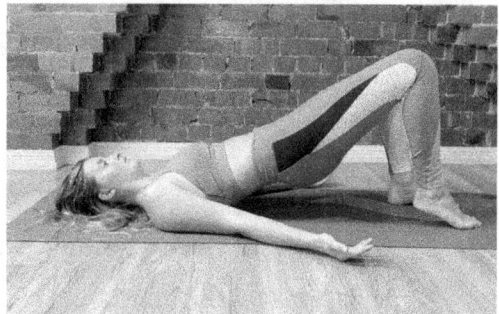

HIP HINGE WITH A ROLLER (FORWARD LEAN)

Generally, when we bend forwards the first 30° of movement should be from the hip joint. Often, we bend only from the lumbar spine, which is okay, but it is inefficient so doing it repeatedly, day in day out, can cause pain for many people. If we can learn how use the core/stabiliser muscles in this position then we can move more efficiently, avoid injury and maintain our posture for extended periods.

We perform a lot of our activities of daily living in a "forward lean" or "hip hinge" position, e.g. leaning over a sink to spit out your toothpaste, chopping vegetables at the kitchen bench, bending to pick something up off the floor. A squat and deadlift rely on the same fundamental movement pattern.

In this forward lean or hip hinge exercise, we simplify the movement and maintain the 30° forward flexion position at the hips. You can then focus on activating the glutes on your forward leg to hold the pelvis position, while you maintain a neutral spinal position. The deep back, neck and tummy muscles are therefore maintaining trunk and head alignment.

Using a roller in the hands adds a little complexity. You can then progress to squats and deadlifts, understanding how to flex and extend at the hips while maintaining a neutral spine.

Set up:
- In standing, feet hip-width apart.
- Knees "soft" (i.e. not fully extended or locked, but not bent).
- Neutral lumbar spine.
- The roller held horizontally with hands on both ends so that at rest, it is in contact with your thighs.

Steps:
1. Take a slightly larger than normal step forward with the right foot, maintaining the middle of your right kneecap in line with your 2nd right toe, and ensure

that as you look down, your right knee stays in behind your right toes.

2. Keep weight into the **right heel** throughout.

3. The heel on the left foot should be lifted so that you are on the ball of this foot.

4. Bend forward from your hips only, by about 30°, and flex your right knee just a little more.

5. In this position, if you looked down, your right shoulder should be over the middle of the right thigh and mid-right foot.

6. Your chin should be gently tucked and your eyes looking toward the floor, about 30cm in front of your foot.

7. Maintain this forward lean position as you slowly raise your arms with the roller to shoulder height and then lower.

8. Repeat shoulder flexion up to 15 times then swap legs and repeat x15. 2-3 sets.

Tips:

- Maintain a neutral lumbar spine and slight shoulder blade contractions throughout.

- Aim for an imaginary straight line (if you were looking side-on) running diagonally through your ear, shoulder and hip (and knee and ankle) when in the forward lean position – in fact perform your exercise side-on to a mirror to assess your alignment.

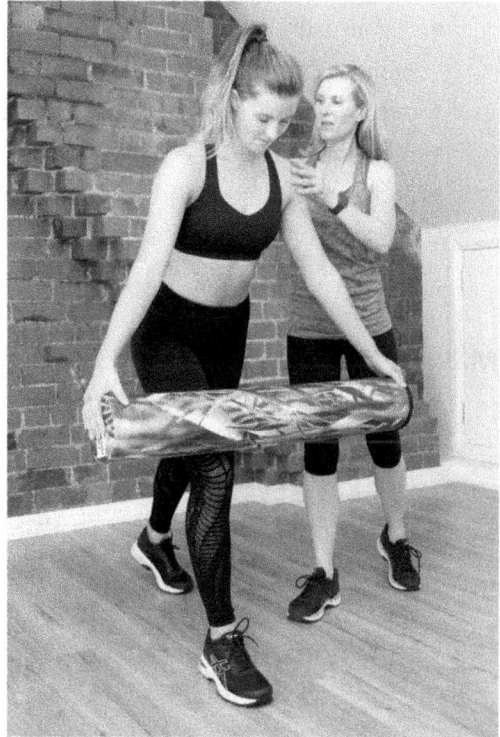

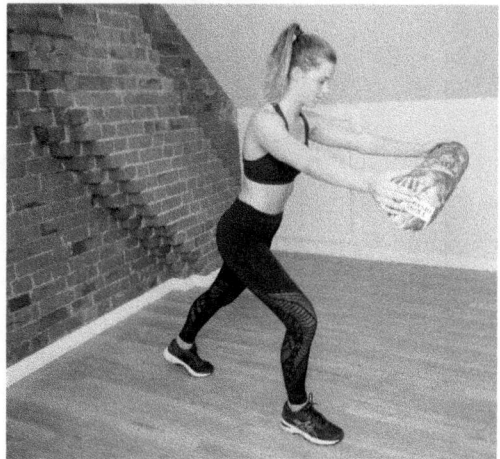

- Maintain your weight into the heel of the forward foot to improve your glute contraction.
- Remember to breathe normally throughout.
- There should be no back pain or fatigue.
- This exercise can be performed in sitting first to make it easier. Either sit on a Swiss ball or sit on the edge of a chair. Feet and knees are hip width apart. Follow the instructions 4-7 as above. Repeat x10-20.

Make it harder:
- Raise the roller above the head without overusing neck muscles, or losing your neutral back.
- Add in trunk rotation to the right and left when in forward lean by moving the roller horizontally to the right, then back to the midline, then to the left.

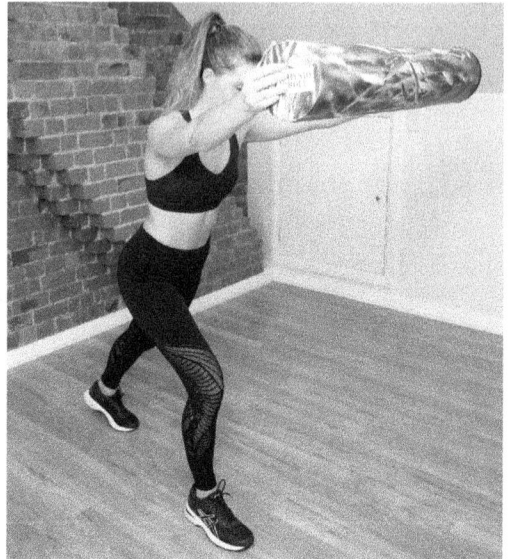

STEP STANCE BALANCE

This is a simple but very effective balance exercise that you can perform with or without shoes.

Set up:
- Stand side-on to a wall (or heavy, stable piece of furniture) within reaching distance.

Steps:
1. Place your right foot directly in front of your left foot, leaving about half a foot's distance in between.
2. Keep your knees slightly flexed, neutral lumbar spine and breathe normally.
3. Maintain for 30+ seconds.
4. Swap feet over and repeat.

Tips:
- You will wobble, but your arms can be lifted out to the sides if you need them to help you balance.

Make it harder:
- Turn your head slowly to the right, then back to the centre, then slowly to the left. Repeat x5. Repeat with the other foot in front.
- Close your eyes and balance for 30+ seconds.
- Close your eyes and turn your head as above.

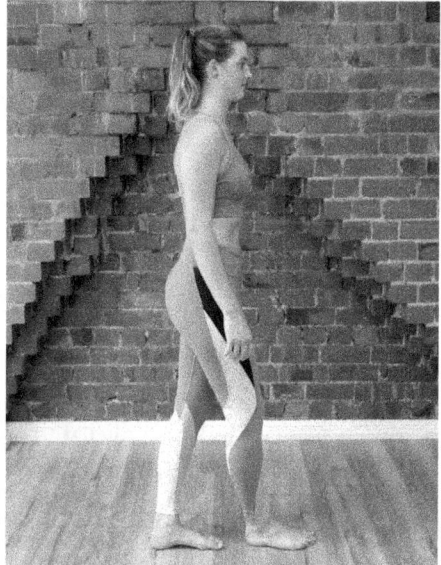

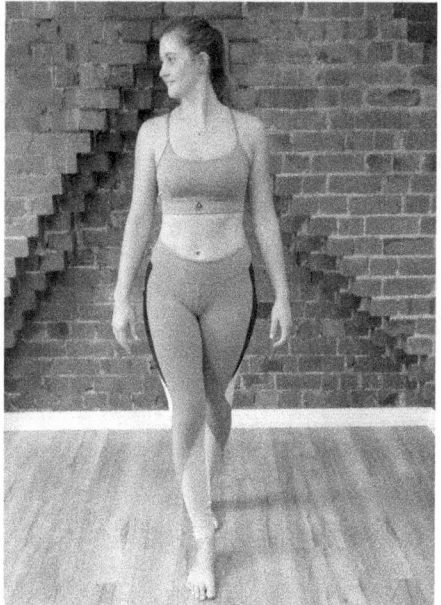

SINGLE LEG BALANCE AND ROLL

This is a basic balance exercise where you have an unstable object underneath one foot that is also elevated. It is designed to get the glutes activated on the standing leg while the foot on the roller moves back and forth.

Set up:
- Place the roller horizontally on the floor about 20-30cm in front of you.
- Stand mid-roller with feet hip-width apart, both knees slightly bent.

Steps:
1. Lift the right foot and place the ball of the foot only on the roller.
2. Roll the roller vigorously back and forth – small oscillations.
3. Keep the knee slightly bent on the standing (left) leg.
4. Hips should be level, lumbar spine neutral.
5. Continue for 1-2 minutes.
6. Repeat with the left foot.

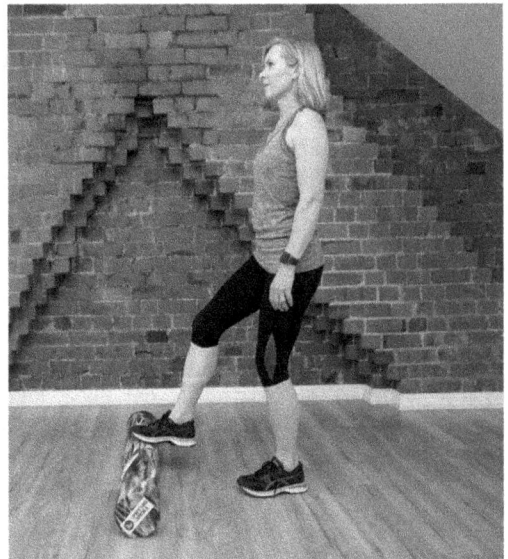

Tips:
- Stand near a wall if your balance is poor; use fingertip support as necessary.
- You should feel your glutes working on the standing leg. Keep weight into the standing leg heel to facilitate this.

Make it harder:
- Close your eyes while continuing to roll the roller.
- Progress to stand on top of the roller with both feet and balance (see roller balance exercise page 88).

MODIFIED BIERING-SORENSON

This is a deep neck strengthening exercise that is performed without a roller. It is a great beginner exercise that helps to strengthen the deep neck extensors in a pain-free position. This exercise can be easily progressed by adding in arm movements.

Set up:
- Face down on the floor, arms by your sides, palms facing up.
- Forehead only resting on a pillow if needed (so that you can breathe).
- Neck and shoulders are relaxed.

Steps:
1. Breathe in and as you breathe out gently tighten the deep tummy, draw your shoulder blades down and back and keeping your chin slightly tucked, lift the forehead from the floor/pillow about 5cm.
2. Pause and then breathe in as you lower back to the floor.
3. Repeat x10.

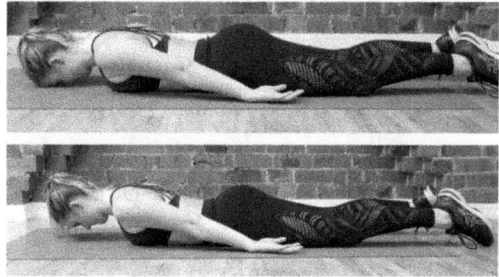

Tips:
- Your shoulders will lift from the floor but not your hands.
- Don't let your chin un-tuck.
- Don't lift your feet.
- You should not feel neck or back pain.

Make it harder:
- Bend the elbows so that they line up with the shoulders with palms facing the floor. Elbows will be in line with the ears. Repeat as above, simultaneously lifting the arms as you lift the head and shoulders from the floor. Repeat x10.

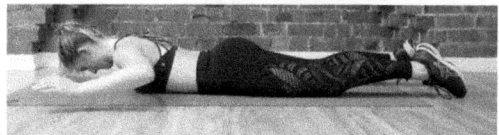

BASIC BIRD DOG

"Bird dog" is a great core exercise that also works the deep stabilising muscles in the neck and at the shoulder blades. It is another exercise that should be mastered at a basic level before introducing a roller.

There are also many beneficial mini movements within this basic 4-point kneeling exercise, such as shoulder blade protraction/retraction in a weight-bearing position and pelvic tilting in kneeling.

Set up:

- On the floor, in kneeling with hands lined up directly under your shoulders, elbows straight but not hyperextended, i.e. elbow creases facing inwards.
- Your hips should be directly over your knees, lumbar spine in a neutral position.
- Keep your neck lengthened, chin slightly tucked and eyes looking to the floor.
- Spread fingers and push hands gently into the floor to turn on the shoulder blade muscles a little.
- Engage your deep tummy muscles gently as well.

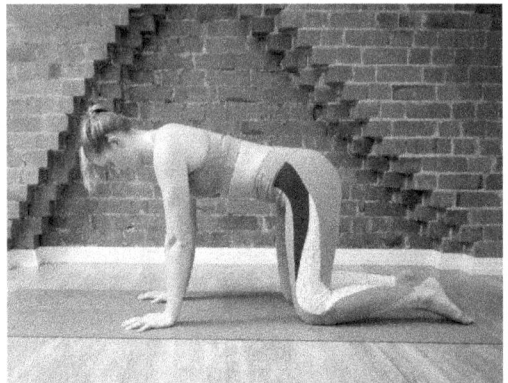

Steps:

1. Take a breath in and as you breathe out, raise your right arm out in front of your right shoulder. Pause, then breathe

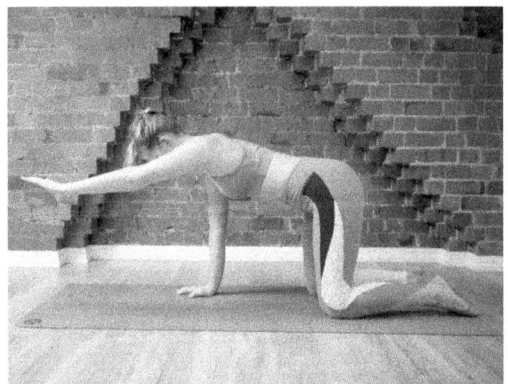

in and return your hand to the floor. Make sure you turn on this right shoulder blade muscle again.

2. Breathe out as you lift the left hand out in front of your left shoulder. Pause. Breath in return as above.
3. Breathe out, slowly extend the right leg so that you straighten the knee but keep your big toe in contact with the floor. Return.
4. Repeat with the left leg. Return.
5. Continue until you have done 4-6 reps (both arm and both leg extensions = 1 rep).

Tips:

- The aim of this exercise is to maintain your neutral back position while your limbs are moving. As you do the leg extensions try to minimise any dropping of your pelvis by sliding your foot out till your knee straightens and then slide back. Don't rush.
- Try a small ball on your lumbar spine to monitor your neutral back position. If you drop or lift too much the ball will roll off.
- There are many variations – you could repeat x4-6 leg extensions on one side then go to x4-6 on the other leg, skipping the arm movements.
- Make sure your knees remain hip-width apart; there is always a tendency to move them closer together.
- Perform this exercise side-on to a mirror so that you can check your alignment.
- Try not to drop the head but ensure the neck is lengthened throughout.
- Knees should not hurt – use a thick mat on the floor if they do.
- If wrists are uncomfortable, try tenting your fingers or using a half roller (semi-circular shape). Alternatively, you could use a very small cushion, sand/rice bag or small, rolled up towel to elevate the wrist.

Make it harder:

- Slide your leg out and then lift your foot from the floor.
- Try extending the opposite leg with the outstretched arm.
- Add in a roller at your hands or feet (page 112 & 114).

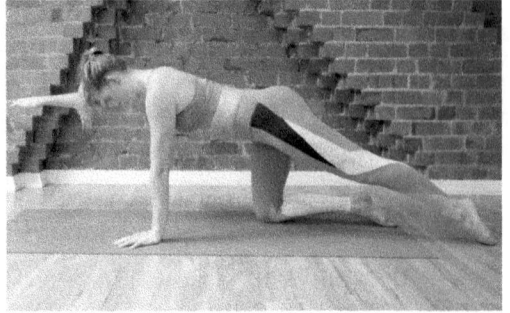

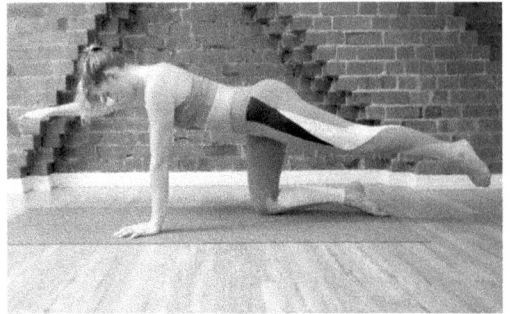

CHIN TUCKS

This is a basic neck exercise that is performed without a roller. Chin tucks help to ease the symptoms associated with a "poke neck" or forward head posture. They help to keep the head aligned on top of the spine. Chin tucks are great to practice every day if you sit at a desk for extended periods.

Set up:
- Chin tucks can be performed in either sitting or standing.
- *In standing:* feet and knees should be hip-width apart, knees soft, with your body weight evenly distributed between the balls and the heels of both feet. Your spine should be in a neutral position, with ears aligned over shoulders.
- *In sitting:* feet and knees should be hip-width apart with lower back supported so that your spine is neutral. Your ears should be aligned with your shoulders.
- Your breathing should be relaxed and down into your diaphragm.
- Bend your right elbow so that your fist rests on your chest with the base of your right thumb resting on your sternum.
- Extend your right index finger so that it just touches your chin.

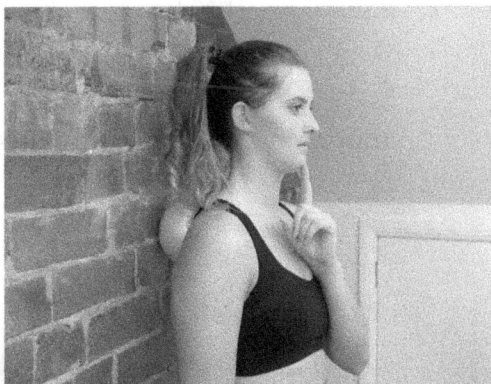

Steps:
1. Gently draw your shoulder blades down and back.
2. Breathe in and as you breathe out move your head and chin straight back, about 2-3cm away from your index finger, lengthening through the back of your neck and keeping your eyes forwards.

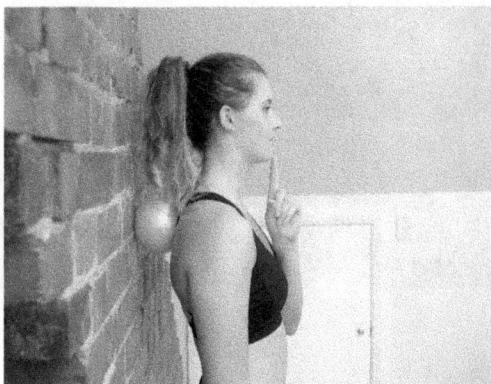

3. You will make a double chin.
4. Pause, breathe in and then relax back to the start position, with your chin touching your index finger.
5. Repeat x10. 1-2 sets.

Tips:

- Try to keep the rest of the body still.
- Your head should move back no more than around 3cm.
- Keep your chin level.
- You can use your small ball on your spine in between your shoulder blades (as pictured above) to encourage a slight shoulder blade contraction and improve your body awareness.

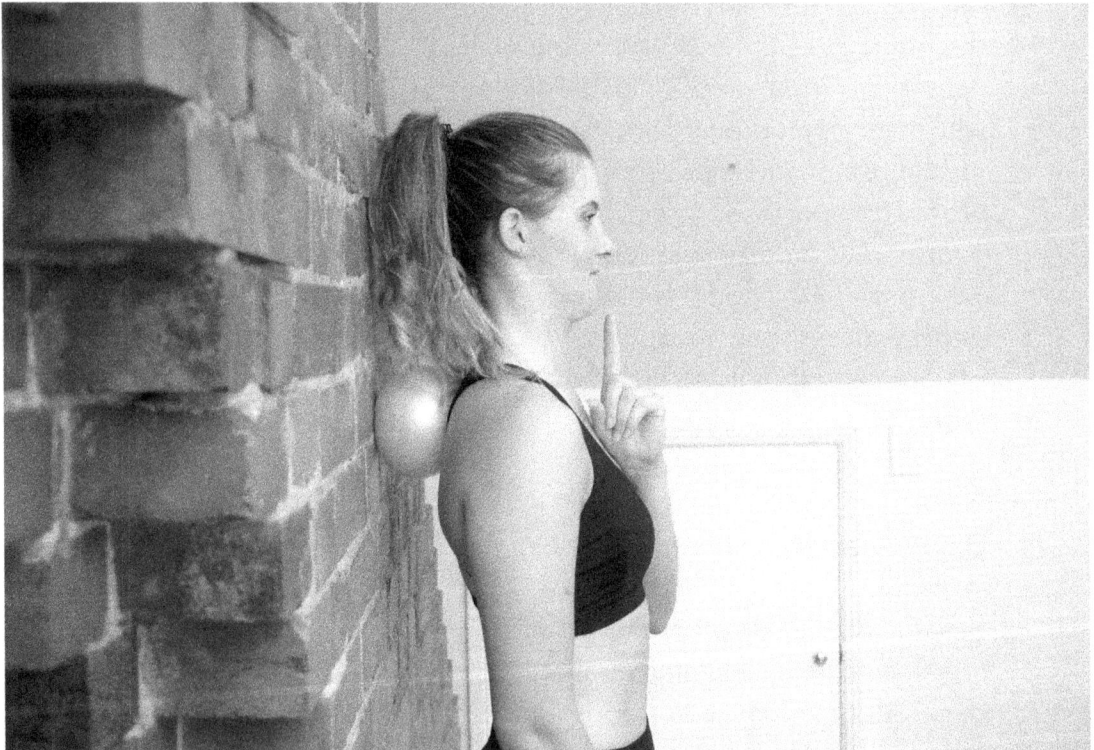

HEAD NODS

Head nods are best performed with a small ball at a wall. The simple repeated chin tuck and roll movement is a great exercise for easing neck pain and improving upper cervical spine mobility. Head nods can also be a great way to ease a headache.

Set up:

- Standing about 10cm from a wall, feet and knees hip-width apart, knees slightly bent, neutral lumbar spine.
- Place your small ball on the wall at forehead level. NB. It should not be completely in front of your eyes.
- Draw your shoulder blade muscles down and back a little.
- Relax your upper neck muscles and shoulders.

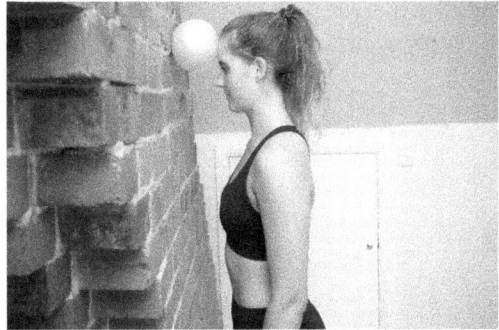

Steps:

1. Make a dent in the ball with your forehead, i.e. push your forehead onto the ball onto the wall at about a 25-50% push.
2. Tuck the chin slightly.
3. Then maintaining the dent in the ball, gently roll your chin towards your chest and slowly return to the start position.
4. It should feel "nice", like it is gently stretching and moving through your neck. There should be no pain.
5. Repeat your head nods x10-20.

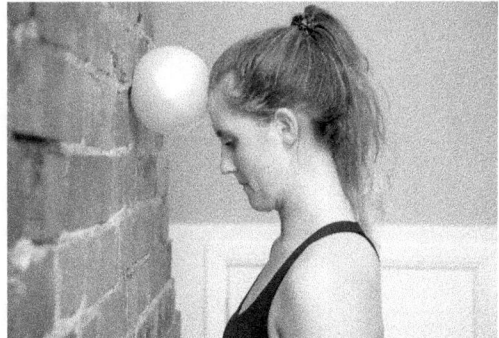

Tips:
- It can often help to imagine a pivot point through your temporomandibular joint (at the jaw); nod through this pivot point.
- Try not to poke your chin when you return to the starting position.
- Maintain the push on the ball throughout.
- The rest of the body should remain still.
- Breathe normally down into your diaphragm throughout.

Make it harder:
- Maintain your push on the ball and rotate your head slowly to the right then slowly rotate to the left; the ball should move from one side of your forehead to the other. Try to keep your chin level throughout.
- Repeat x5 each side. 2 sets.

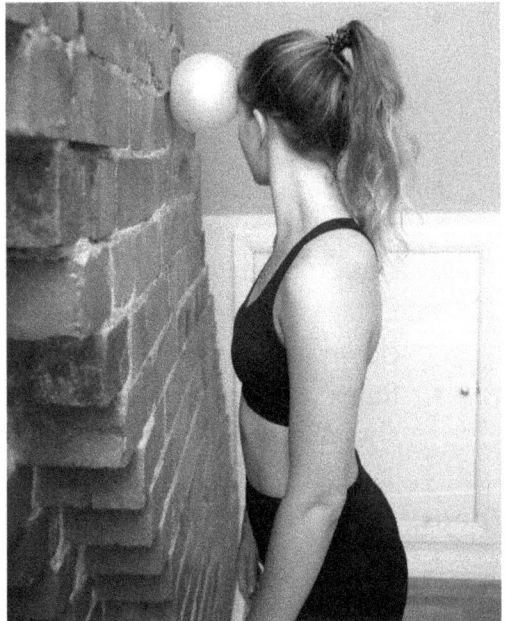

CHAPTER 5

Now You're on a Roll

"Practice puts brains into your muscles."
Sam Snead

By now you will have mastered a few of the basic movement patterns (squat, hinge, push) in a simplified way. You will have also figured out where your core muscles are and how they work. You are now ready to add a little more complexity with these intermediate exercises.

ROLLER SQUAT

A basic squat is a popular strength exercise that targets the thighs (quads and hamstrings), glutes and your core – all at once.

Squats are also one of the most commonly performed movements that you do daily – you do a squat-type action every time you lower your bottom into a chair, onto a lounge or onto a toilet! You squat to grab your shoes, the coin you dropped on the floor or the wet towel the kids left on the tiles.

But do you cringe at the thought of doing squats? Do you lower your body gingerly down into a chair, using the arm rests because your knees hurt and creak?

Squats, by strengthening your quads and glutes, help to improve the function of knees and hips, ankles and spines. Squatting with correct form requires a degree of stabilisation from the core. This is increased when you add in weights. In this way squats are really helpful for helping you to remain mobile for longer and perform your daily activities with less pain.

This free-standing squat is a step up from the wall version presented in the rookie section because you need to maintain your neutral lumbar spine position without external feedback. Despite being a simple movement, it is important to learn the correct form. A sumo squat position is described below (because it is often easier to do) but there are many squat variations (see page 82).

Set up:
- Standing, feet wider than knees, knees wider than hips.
- Feet pointing out at 1 and 11 o'clock.
- The centre of each of your kneecaps should line up with your 2nd toe.
- Lumbar spine neutral.
- Hands at each end of your roller; roller lightly resting (horizontally) on your thighs.

Steps:

1. Breathe in and then breathe out as you slowly bend your hips and knees and move your bottom down and back. Keep your weight into your heels and your lumbar spine neutral as you lower your bottom towards the floor.
2. *Move in the range that is comfortable for you.*
3. Simultaneously lift the roller out in front, up to chest height.
4. Your kneecaps should be tracking in line with your 2nd toes.
5. Lower the roller as you breathe in, straighten your knees and hips and return to your starting position.
6. Repeat x15-20. 2-3 sets.

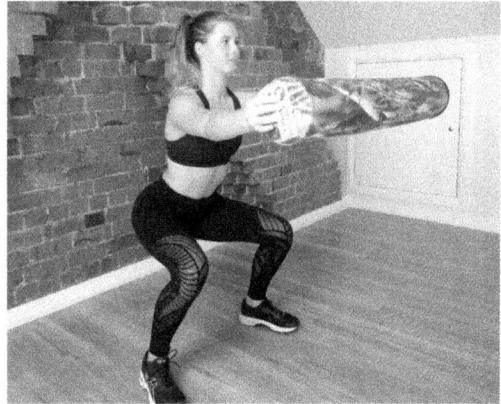

Tips:

- As you squat, maintain your knee alignment and don't let your knees bend past your toes (in the vertical plane), or move towards each other or outwards.
- Keep your weight into your heels throughout your roller squat.
- Maintain a neutral lower back position throughout to avoid "buttwink" (when the pelvis tilts posteriorly at the lower range of the squat, causing the lumbar spine to round and go into flexion).
- Keep your gaze level and try not to poke your chin.
- Your neck should be relaxed, using your shoulder blades to stabilise at your shoulder.
- Do not push into knee pain or back pain. Limit your range to avoid pain.

Make it harder:
- Lift the roller above your head (but don't lose your neutral spine alignment).
- Perform a split squat (or lunge), lowering the rear knee as you lift the roller x10 each leg. 2-3 sets.
- See the Physio on a Roll website for more instructions and variations.

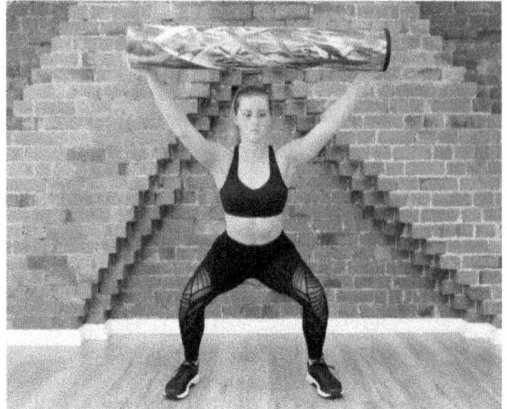

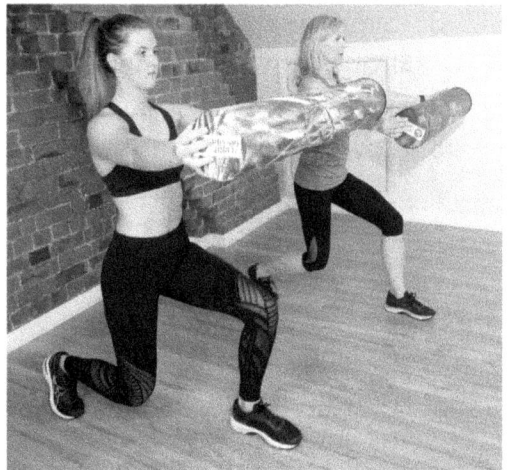

LUNGE WITH A ROLLER – ROTATIONS

Lunges, also known as split squats, are a great exercise for your quads, glutes and core. This is a static lunge exercise that is one of my favourites because the addition of a roller adds to the challenge for your core and your balance. There are a few variations described below.

NB. I often see lunges performed without regard to knee and hip alignment. Poor alignment means that you are less likely to engage your glutes and more likely to experience unnecessary knee pain. As such the instructions below are quite detailed. Follow the cues and try to do your lunge with a roller in front of a mirror, at least initially, to maximise your performance.

Set up:

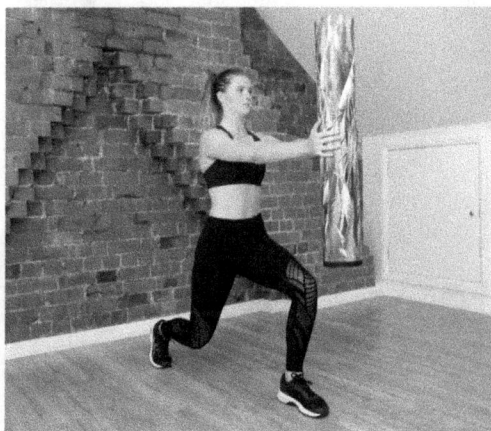

- In standing, feet hip-width apart, roller held vertically in your hands.
- Hands should be mid-roller, opposite each other, positioned below shoulder height, elbows straight and shoulder blades slightly contracted.
- Take a large step forward with your *left* foot.
- Then lift your *right* heel so that you are on the ball of your *right* foot.
- Keep your hips level and both kneecaps aligned with your 2nd toes.
- Keep weight into your *left* (front) heel, but ensure that your *left* knee doesn't move past your *left* big toe.
- A side-on view would show your ear in line with your shoulder, hips and back knee.

Steps

1. Maintain weight into the *left* (front) heel, and level hips.
2. Bend both knees so that you lower the right (back) knee further towards the floor; the front thigh will become more horizontal. Ensure that the front knee doesn't move beyond the toes.
3. Maintain this lunge position.
4. Then breathe in and as you breathe out slowly rotate the roller and upper body towards the left (to about 10 o'clock if we use a clock analogy). Breathe in and rotate slowly back to the starting position.
5. Breathe out as you slowly rotate the roller and your body to the right (to 2 o'clock). Return.

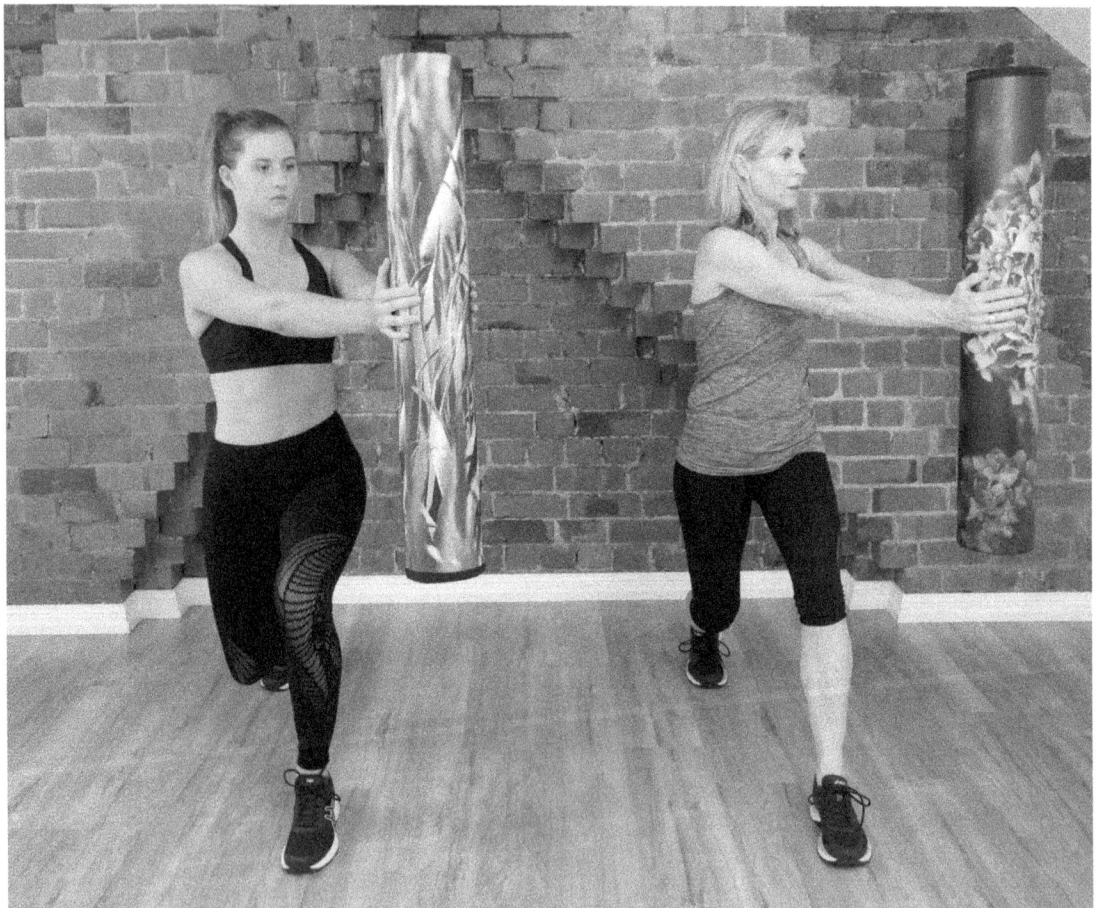

6. Think about keeping your sternum lined up with the roller.
7. Keep alternating the sides. Repeat x10.
8. Change your legs over.
9. Repeat x10. 2-3 sets.

Tips:

- You should feel your glutes on the front leg working hard as well as your quads on the back leg. Your abdominals will be working as well as your shoulders. Your front ankle will wobble a little to help with balance.
- Keep hips level and facing forward throughout. Basically, your torso is twisting on a fixed pelvis.
- Your head can follow your hands or you can maintain your gaze forward and keep your head still as your torso moves.
- Keep your neck and shoulders relaxed.
- If your neck feels uncomfortable, lower your hands and therefore your roller a little. If your neck is still sore, bend your elbows to bring the roller closer to your body and turn your shoulder blades on more.
- Weight into the front heel will help to keep your glutes on and help with your balance.

Make it harder:

- Lower further down into the lunge.
- Rise up and then lower down after each rotation.
- Progress to the advanced roller lunge in the "High Rollers" section (page 127).
- Swap the roller for a weight.

ROLLER HOPS (LOW IMPACT)

Roller hops are a low impact or gentler version of an advanced roller jump exercise. Jumping is something that we used to do easily and often as children, without a thought about how or why. As we age we tend to jump less and less. This might be because jumping requires a strong core and legs and the ability to conjure up explosive power from within.

Research also tells us that we need impact stressors (such as jumps and hops) to promote and maintain our bone density; simple weight-bearing activities such as walking are not enough. Our bodies also get used to the same stimuli all the time so we need to shake it up with different exercises (27).

Please be sure to proceed with caution if your balance or eyesight is poor or if you are osteoporotic.

Set up:
- Place your roller on the floor/ground. Ensure you are on a stable, non-slippery surface, with plenty of space around you and preferably with sneakers on.
- Stand beside your roller, side-on, about halfway along its length.
- Feet about hip-width apart.

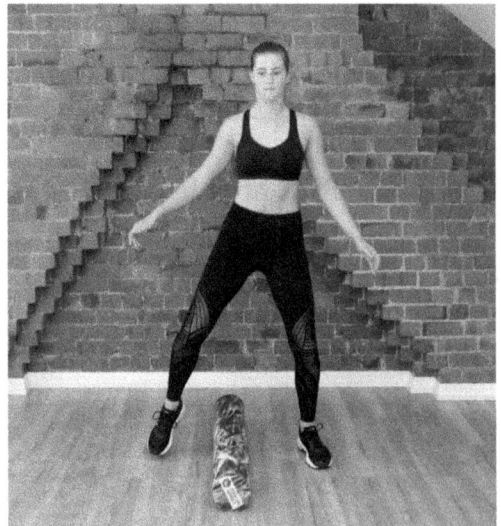

Steps:
1. Bend your knees and hips and with a slight spring, step the foot which is closest to the roller, over the roller, placing first the ball of the foot and then the heel on the floor.
2. Your other foot should follow in quick succession as the first foot touches the floor.

Let it Roll

3. Step back over.
4. Perform sets of 20-30 low impact roller hops over 1-2 minutes.

Tips:
- If this is too intense or difficult, simply step over the roller. As you are able, progress to the "springing" version.
- Try not to look down as you are doing your roller hops.
- If you accidentally touch your roller, stop, make sure you re-align it then start hopping again.
- Use your arms for balance and momentum.

Make it harder:
- Speed up your steps so that the second foot only has the ball of the foot touching the floor before it returns back to the other side of the roller.
- Stand front-on to your roller and step one foot over it, then the other. Then step back over the roller, without turning, then follow with the other foot. Repeat x20-30. 2-3 sets.
- Intersperse low impact with a few roller jumps as in "High Rollers" (page 125).

ROLLER BALANCE

The roller, as a cylindrical object, is a great unstable surface on which you can challenge your balance. Perform this exercise with or without shoes.

Set up:
- Standing beside a wall (or a stable, heavy piece of furniture) with your roller placed perpendicular to the wall/furniture (this is easier than the set up depicted in the photo).
- You should be within an arms distance of the wall/furniture.

Steps:
1. Using the wall for support, carefully step one foot and then the other onto the middle of the roller.
2. Feet should be hip-width apart, knees slightly flexed.
3. Relax the neck and shoulders and try to maintain a neutral lumbar spine.
4. Do try to let go of the wall.
5. Balance for up to 1-2 minutes.

Tips:
- Barefoot will seem easier as your foot will naturally contour around the roller.
- You will wobble, that is normal, as your body tries to maintain your balance.

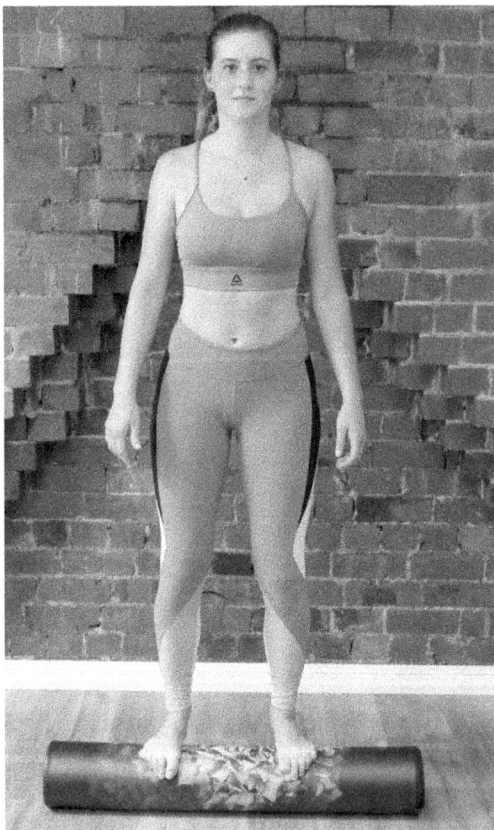

Make it harder:

- Move your roller parallel to the wall as shown in the photos.
- Lower into a small squat and return x10-15.
- Lift one foot off so that you are doing single leg balance on the roller.

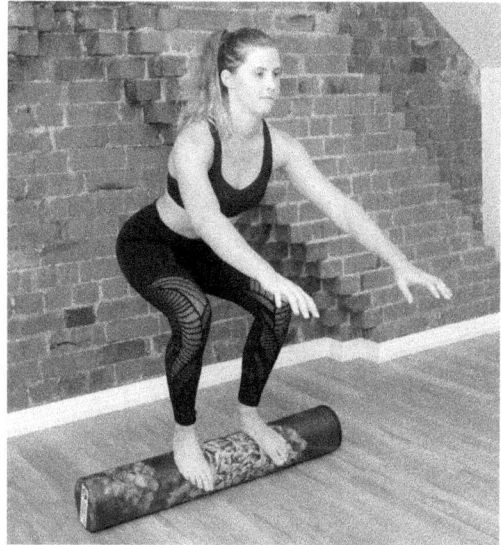

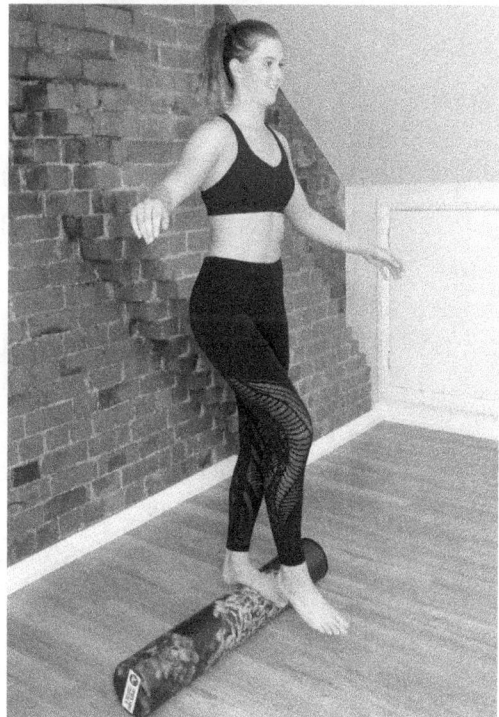

SINGLE KNEE LIFT AND TAP

This exercise works the core as well as the upper and lower body and will also challenge your balance.

Set up:
- In standing, feet hip-width apart, knees slightly flexed.
- Roller resting on your thighs, hands positioned at each end.
- Neck and shoulders relaxed, lumbar spine neutral.

Steps:
1. Lift the roller out in front of your body, arms at around 40° of forward flexion (as shown in the photo) or midway between your belly button and sternum.
2. Maintain this position with shoulder blades drawn down and back a little.
3. Breathe in and as you breathe out lift your right knee towards the roller (about hip height), then lower the leg and stretch it back behind you, around 30cm to tap the floor with your toes.
4. Lift again and repeat x10.
5. Repeat with the left leg x10. 2-3 sets.

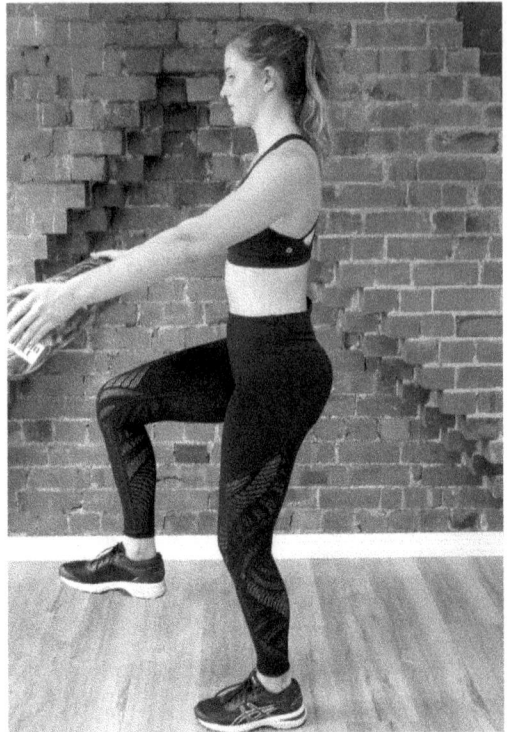

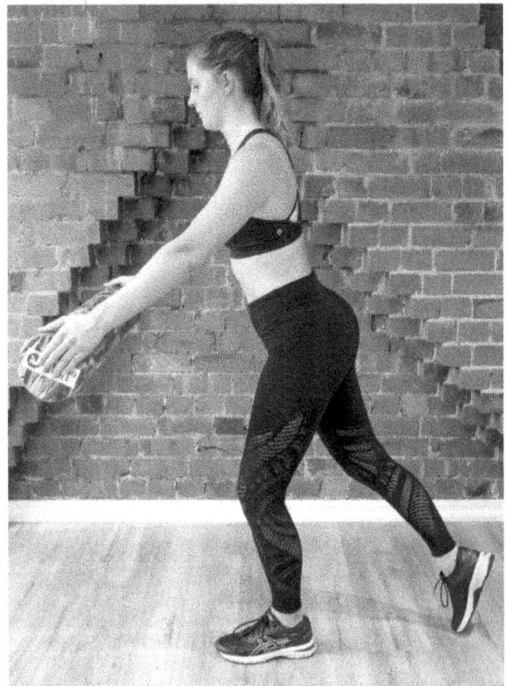

Tips:

- Keep the knee slightly flexed on the standing leg and weight into the heel on the standing leg to help with your balance.
- Your glutes on the standing leg should be working hard.

Make it harder:

- Lift the knee and then lunge that leg further behind you – you will need to bend the standing knee and bend at the hip to allow this and will end up in a hip hinge posture. Repeat x10-15. 2-3 sets.

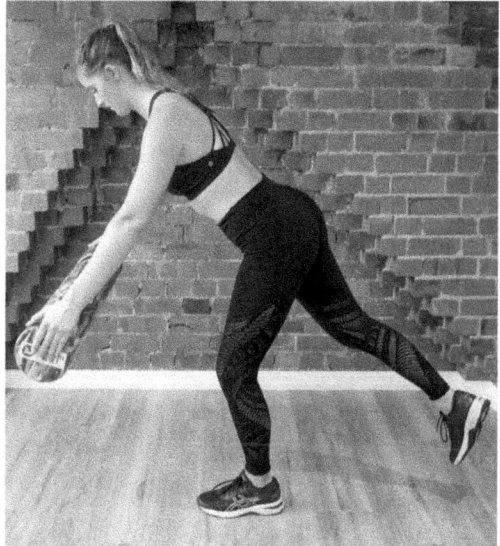

TRICEPS WALL PUSH-UP WITH A ROLLER

This push-up variation is great for those people who tend to overuse their upper neck muscles as the arms are positioned lower on the roller on the wall. It is also easier to engage your shoulder blades. You should feel your shoulders and triceps working hard.

Set up:
- Standing, facing a wall, about an arms-length from the wall.
- Feet and knees hip-width apart and your feet flat on the floor and parallel.
- Place the roller vertically on the wall, the top of the roller aligned *(more or less)* with your forehead.
- Then place your right hand in the middle third of the roller. It should be just below right shoulder height, thumb on one side, fingers on the other.
- Place your left hand about a hands-width below this, again with your thumb on one side and fingers on the other.
- Your elbows should be straight, or slightly bent *(if you suffer from neck pain)* and drawn close to each other.
- Lumbar spine is neutral.

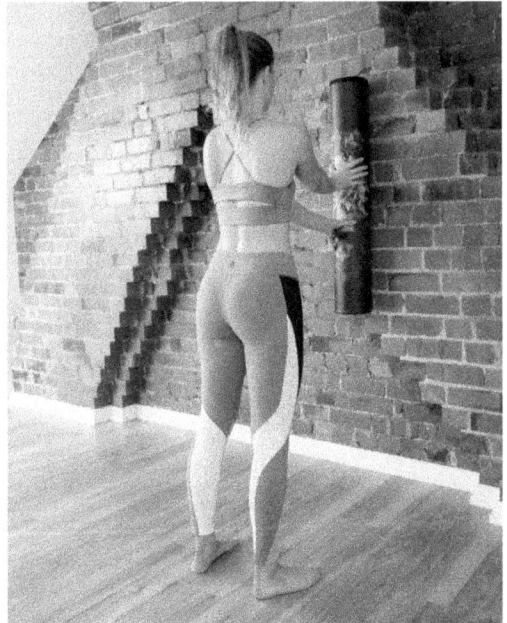

Steps:
1. Gently squeeze shoulder blade muscles down and back a little, by leaning your body weight through your straight arms onto the roller, onto the wall.
2. Maintaining your shoulder blade contractions and pressure through the roller onto the wall, breathe in and bend your elbows, keeping them close together and lower your body, *plank-like*, towards the roller.

3. Move in the range that you can manage.
4. Breathe out as you return to the arms straight position.
5. Repeat x10.
6. Swap your hands over so that the left hand is now uppermost and repeat x10.
7. Perform 2-3 sets with a break in between.

Tips:

- Try not to let your head drop or move forward of your body. Maintain a slight chin tuck.
- Your hips should not sag forward.
- Keep your upper neck muscles relaxed. You should only feel your shoulders and upper arms working hard.
- If your neck is activated, stand closer to the wall, with more elbow flexion, and perform the exercise in a smaller range.
- Try to maintain your pressure on the roller on the wall to prevent it sliding down the wall.
- Make sure that the top hand remains at or slightly below shoulder height.

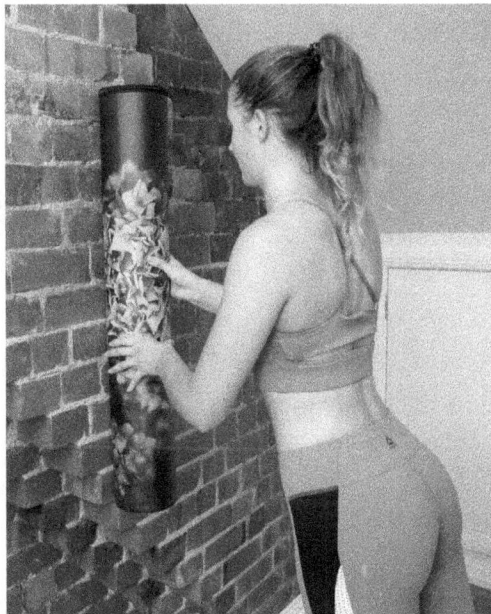

Make it harder:

- Rise up on your toes and perform your triceps exercise as described above.
- Rise up on your toes and then extend one leg behind you, from the hip, maintaining your neutral lumbar spine. Repeat your push-up as above. Then repeat with the other leg extended.
- Perform a single arm triceps push-up with your hand placed mid-roller and both feet on the floor but on your toes.
- Try triceps with weights (page 108) in a supine lying position on the roller.

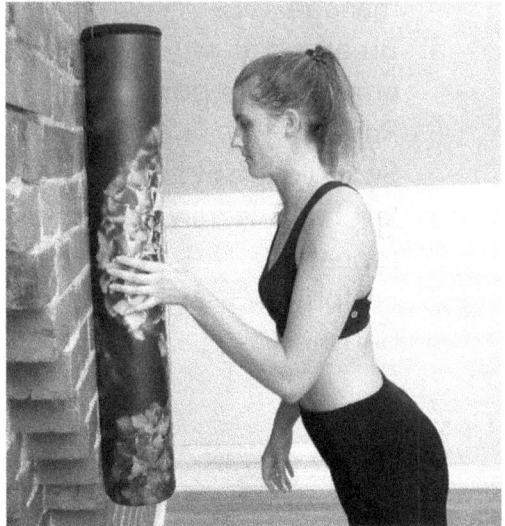

BRIDGE WITH A ROLLER

This bridging variation is useful for lumbar spine mobility and upper body awareness. You will also notice a thoracic spine longitudinal massage which can improve thoracic mobility and in turn benefit stiff necks and increase shoulder range of motion. It can be easily progressed through to an advanced exercise.

Set up:
- Supine on the roller in basic set up position (see page 41).
- Feet could be a little closer to the end of the roller (to help with glute recruitment).

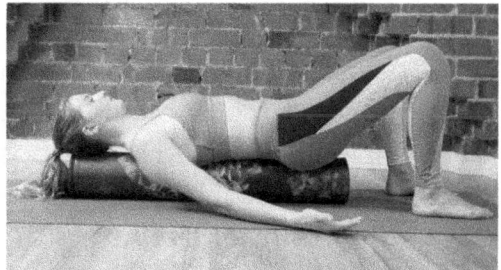

Steps:
1. Breathe out and tilt pelvis so that lower back flattens towards the roller, and squeeze your bottom.
2. Then gently push into your heels and roll your body up off the roller, one vertebra at a time, lifting your pelvis until your hips are aligned with your knees and shoulders (side view). Keep squeezing your bottom.
3. Pause, and breathe in as you return to your starting position by slowly lowering your spine one vertebrae at a time back onto the roller. Relax.
4. Repeat x10. 2-3 sets.

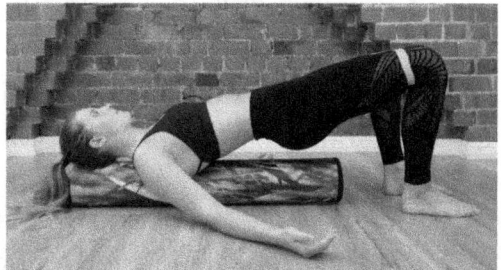

Tips:
- You should not feel your hamstrings (backs of thighs) or lower back working at all; bring your feet slightly closer to the end of the roller if you are having difficulty turning off your hamstrings.
- Make sure your neck and shoulders remain relaxed throughout; turn the palms of your hands towards the ceiling if your neck wants to turn on.

- Try to keep your pelvis level.
- Don't lift your hips too high, arch through the thoracic spine or "pop" your ribs.
- NB. You will move through a smaller range than a bridge performed on the floor because you are elevated 15cm off the floor via the roller.

Make it harder:
- Use only elbow support on the floor.
- Cross your arms across chest (i.e. no arm support on the floor).
- Hold the elevated bridge position for 5-10 seconds before lowering.
- Maintain an elevated bridge position and perform alternating heel lifts x3-5 reps each side.
- Add a resistance band at your knees and do bent knee fallouts (either bilateral or unilateral) in a bridge position x3-5 reps. 2-3 sets.
- Do a single leg bridge on the roller (push up with both feet on the floor, then lift one knee over your hip and hold, lower and then repeat on the other side before lowering back down to the roller). Do 3-5 sets.
- See the *Physio on a Roll* website for more options.

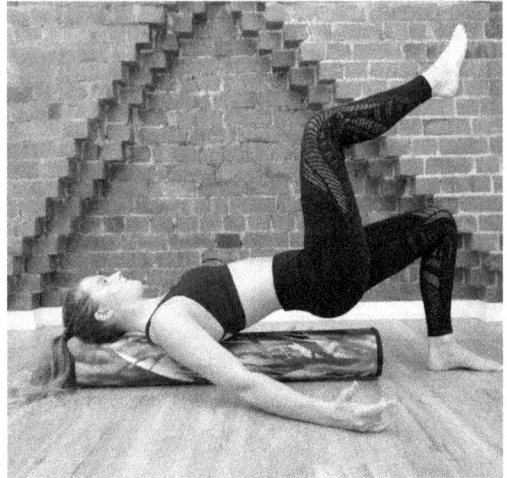

ABDOMINALS – ROLLER OVERHEAD

A simple version of this exercise was introduced in Roller Rookies. It can be easily modified to suit the individual, to make it easier or harder by changing the leg position and/or the number of repetitions. I use this exercise frequently in classes, as a series; beginning with a single static knee over the hip, then moving the knee, then both knees static over the hips.

Set up:

- Supine lying on a flat surface, with knees bent, feet and knees hip-width apart.
- Neutral lumbar spine.
- Chin slightly tucked, neck lengthened with your head on or off a pillow as desired.
- Roller raised over your chest so that your hands on the ends of the roller align with the shoulders.

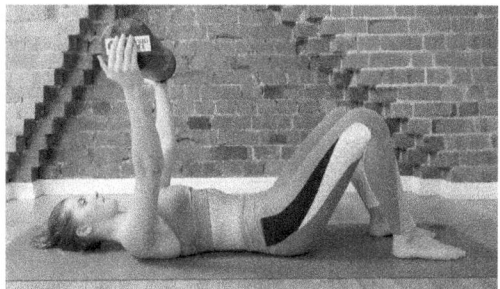

Steps:

1. Maintaining your neutral lumbar spine, breathe in then breathe out and raise your right knee over your right hip.
2. Maintain the right knee position as you breathe out and lower the roller behind your head towards the floor.
3. Breathe in and return the roller to the starting position where your hands are over your shoulders.
4. Repeat the roller behind the head x10.

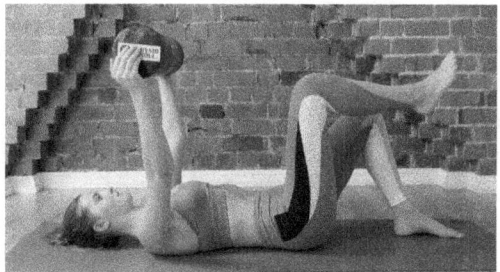

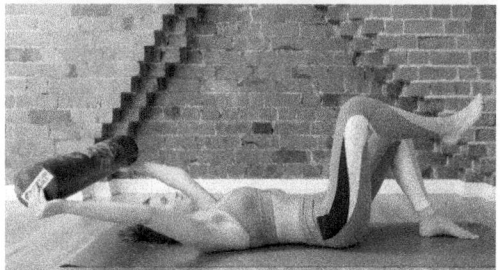

5. Then lower your right foot back to the floor.
6. Repeat with the left knee over left hip as above x10.

Tips:
- Relax the neck and shoulders, i.e. try to let your shoulders "roll" in their sockets and try not to let them creep up towards your ears.
- Try not to let your ribs "pop", i.e. keep your thoracic spine lengthened and rib cage flat.
- Your spine should not arch or flatten as your arms move. Contract your deep tummy muscles at a low level if you need to so that your lumbar spine stays in a neutral position.
- You should lightly touch the floor with your roller on the first repetition only, so you know where the floor is. The following reps should stop just short of the floor.
- There should be no back pain, neck pain or pulling. If your back hurts, reassess your neutral position. You can place a small pillow in your lower back area for support if necessary. Alternatively go back to an easier abdominal exercise such as single knee lift.

Make it harder:
- Raise the right knee over the right hip and then extend/straighten your right knee towards the floor while simultaneously lowering the roller behind your head. Repeat x10. Then repeat with the left leg x10.

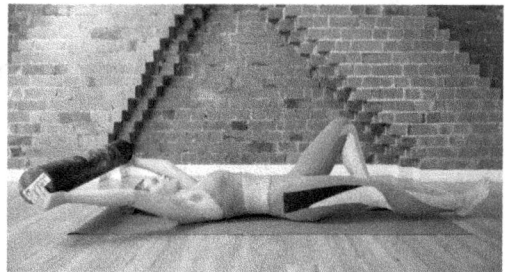

- Breathe in and raise the right knee over the right hip as you breathe out. Then, with the next breath out, raise the left knee over the left hip. Keep the knees stationary in the air as you breathe out and lower the roller towards the floor. Breathe in

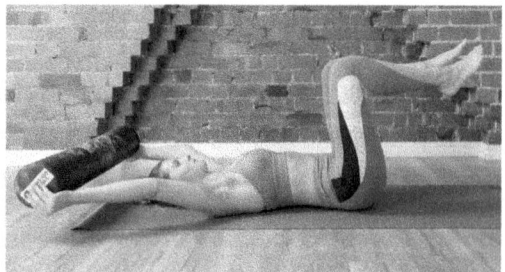

and return to the position over the shoulders. Breathe out and lower the roller again and continue for 3-5 reps. Lower one foot to the floor and then the other. Have a small rest and then repeat x3-5 sets. NB. When you raise both knees over your hips your back will flatten a little more towards the floor. Don't arch it or press into the floor, just try to maintain the slightly flatter position when you take the roller behind your head.

- See advanced abdominals roller overhead (Physio on a Roll website).

ABDOMINALS – DEAD BUG

Moving the opposite arm and leg is an abdominal exercise classically known as a "dead bug". Adding a roller, with its inherent instability and the long lever actions of the exercise, effectively works the core.

Set up:

- Supine on the roller, basic set up position.
- Place your right hand over your right shoulder, with your palm facing in towards the body.
- Place your left knee over your left hip.
- Your left forearm is on the floor for support.
- Lumbar spine is neutral.

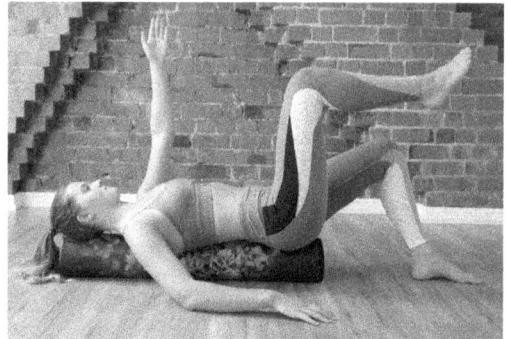

Steps:

1. Breathe in and as you breathe out slowly straighten and lower the left leg towards the floor while simultaneously taking the right arm behind the head toward the floor (elbow straight).
2. Move the arm and leg until they are parallel with the floor, but don't touch the floor.
3. Breathe in and move the arm and leg (by bending the knee) simultaneously, back to the starting position.
4. Repeat x10, with this arm and leg combination.
5. Swap carefully to the opposite arm and leg and repeat x10. 2-3 sets.

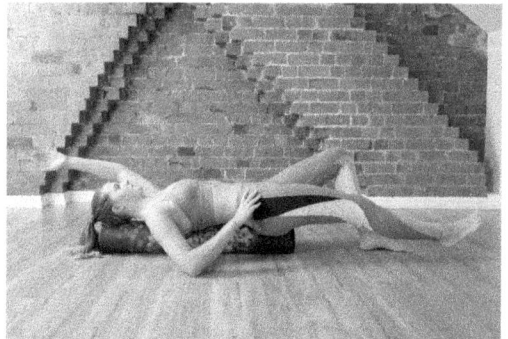

Tips:

- *One side (of opposite arm and leg) will be always seem to be easier to perform, compared to the other. Practice makes your dead bug perfect.*
- The shoulder should roll within its socket; you should not feel the shoulder being elevated toward your ear by overusing your neck muscles. Do not move into any pain, stop short of pain if you find your shoulder is uncomfortable.
- The front of the thigh on the moving leg will start to feel uncomfortable because you are doing a repeated straight leg raise action. It is simply running out of "fuel" and will feel better when you stop and swap sides.
- Make sure that when you do swap legs, you go slowly and maintain your neutral lumbar spine and place the foot back on the floor aligned with the hip of that leg to maintain your base of support. It should not be too close to the end of the roller either.
- Relax the neck throughout the exercise.
- Your lumbar spine should not hurt, lift or flatten while the arm and leg are moving.
- Keep your kneecap and toes pointing directly up toward the ceiling as you bend and straighten to minimise knee pain.

Make it harder:

- Progress your dead bug by using only elbow support on the floor.
- Progress to no arm support on the floor and the non-moving hand resting lightly on the tummy.
- Increase the repetitions to x15-20 each side.
- Add in a small hand weight (1kg) to the moving arm.

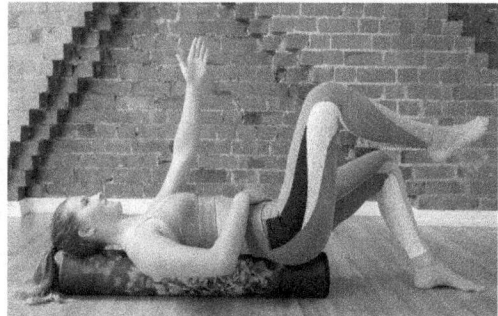

SIT-UP ON A ROLLER

The sit-up or "crunch" is given a makeover on the roller, working all of your abdominals and massaging the thoracic spine simultaneously. Using a high resistance thera-band supports the head and reduces the tendency in a crunch to just use the strong anterior neck muscles (your sternocleidomastoids) when you lift. This technique helps you to avoid neck strain and teaches you how to "let go" of the neck while you also strengthen the deep anterior neck muscles. You will also work your triceps.

There are videos available on the *Physio on a Roll* website that demonstrate this exercise if you are new to this technique or need more help.

NB. If you dislike the band, or find it difficult to manage or achieve the desired neck relaxation, simply use your hands interlaced behind your head for support. Keep your elbows in line with your ears, chin tucked and push into your hands with your head as you lift your head.

Set up:
- Supine lying on top of the roller, basic set up.
- Place a heavy resistance thera-band, **flat** (not scrunched up) around the back of the head.
- The ends of the band should be in each hand, and you should be holding the band about 20cm from each end (assuming your band is around 1.2-1.5 metres long).

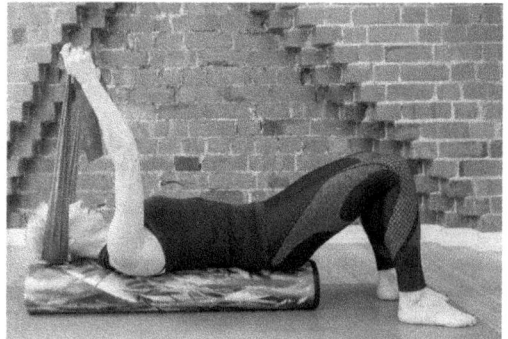

- Pull on the band quite firmly, extending both elbows so they are just short of being straight. The pull is important as this supports the weight of your head in the band.
- Make sure your wrists are also straight and that palms are facing each other.

Steps:

1. Tuck the chin a little and lift head from the roller a little, making sure that the band holds the weight of the head.
2. Maintaining your arm position as above, use your stomach muscles to slowly lift/curl your ribcage towards your belly button.
3. Then slowly and gently lower back down towards the roller, just stopping short of touching the roller.
4. Breathe out as you lift.
5. Breathe in as you lower.
6. Repeat x15-20. Do 2-3 sets with a rest in between.

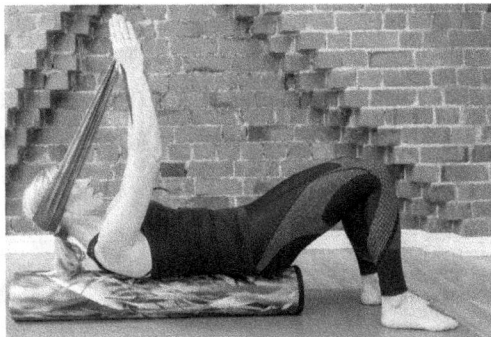

Tips:

- Lift in the range that is comfortable for you – try not to pull on the head with the band, focus on your stomach muscles lifting you. Your arms don't change their position or lift your head.
- Try to relax the neck and shoulders. Your neck should not hurt. You should feel your abdominals working, especially near your lower ribs.
- Keep your wrists straight and palms facing each other throughout with your elbows just off full extension – if they bend too much your arms will begin to fatigue.
- Maintain a gentle chin tuck throughout – don't poke your chin.

Make it harder:
- Lift one knee over the hip and hold in that position while you perform your sit-up.
- Add in a diagonal movement to target the obliques, i.e. aim both hands (still shoulder-width apart) towards the outside of one knee. Either repeat to that side or alternate sides. Repeat x10-15. 3 sets.

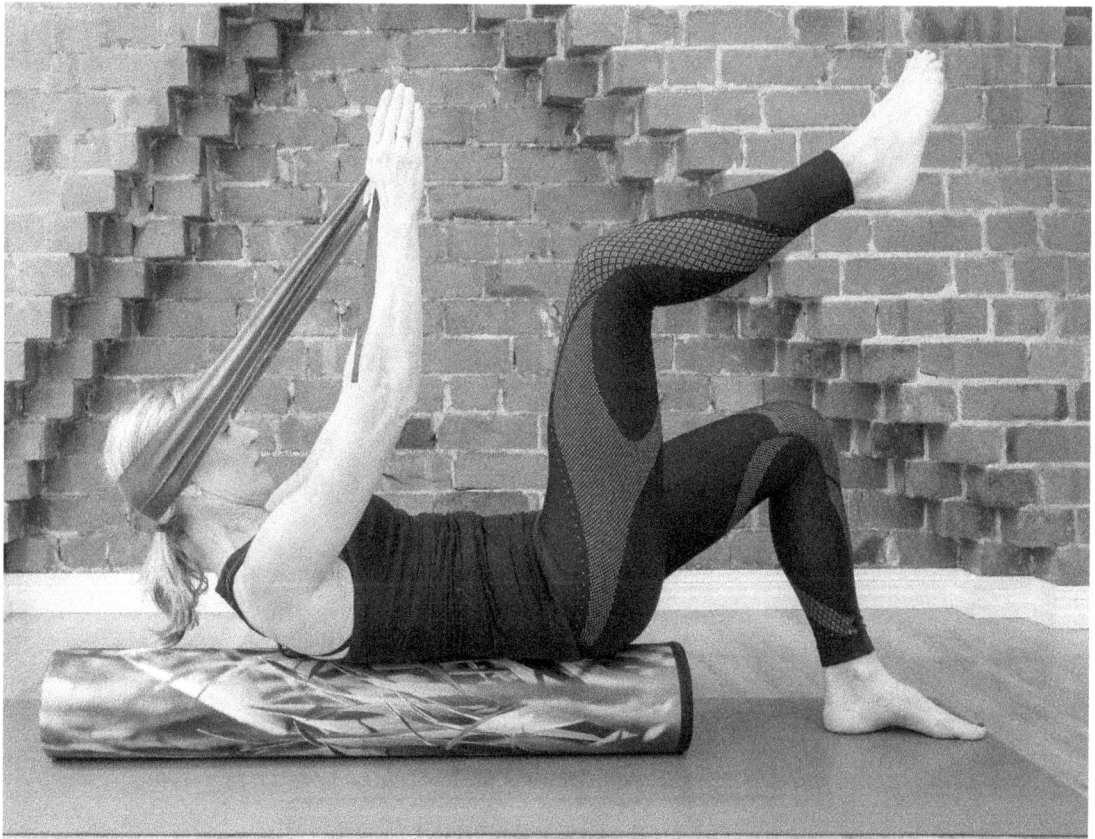

ABDOMINALS – SINGLE KNEE THEN DOUBLE KNEE LIFT

This is a harder abdominal exercise where both feet are off the ground at one point. As such you need to be aware of what is happening to your lower back and your breathing.

Set up:
- Supine on the roller in basic set up position.

Steps:
1. Inhale, then exhale and slowly lift the right knee over the right hip.
2. Inhale, then exhale and slowly lift the left knee over the left hip.
3. Slowly lower right foot to the floor.
4. Then lower left foot to the floor.
5. Repeat, this time starting with left leg.
6. Keep alternating the start leg.
7. Your breathing will become timed with the leg movements.
8. Repeat x10. 2-3 sets.

Tips:
- Don't let lumbar spine arch or squash into the roller, especially as the 2nd leg lifts. It will be flatter on the roller than your normal neutral position – just maintain this.
- There should be no back pain.
- Relax your neck and shoulders.
- Ribs should not "pop".
- Keep your breathing normal and it will be in time with each leg movement after the initial lift.

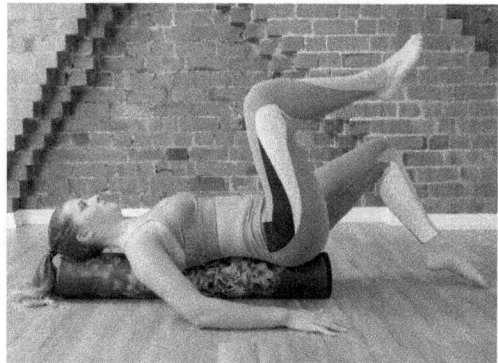

Make it harder:
- Go to elbow support only on the floor.
- Increase the reps.

BENCH PRESS ON A ROLLER

Bench press is a functional exercise as it replicates a pushing action. Performed on a roller it will effectively work the core, shoulders, upper arms and chest.

I use bench press on a roller as part of a program to ease neck pain with my clients. It allows you to improve your upper body strength while the head and neck are supported on the roller and you can feel the shoulder blades engaging. Often you may be able to use heavier weights in this position than the weights you use in a standing exercise.

Set up:
- Supine lying on your roller as per basic set up.
- Weights in each hand, your palms facing your feet, your elbows bent lower than shoulder height so that your weights rest near your armpits.
- Your shoulder blade muscles should be slightly contracted.

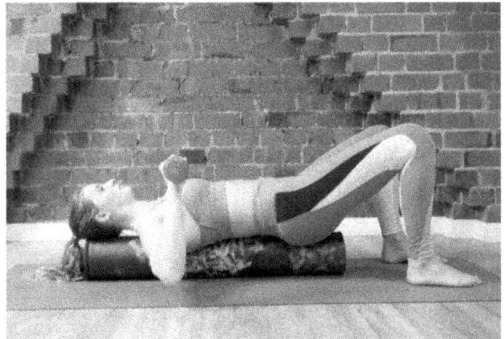

Steps:
1. Breathe in and as you breathe out slowly straighten your elbows and push the weights towards the ceiling, keeping them in line with the chest.
2. Breathe in, bend your elbows and return to the start position, but don't let your elbows touch the floor.
3. Repeat x10-15. 2-3 sets.

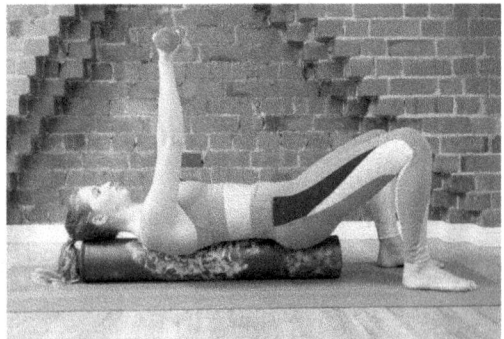

Tips:

- Make sure your ribs don't "pop", i.e. thoracic spine should stay in contact with roller and breathing should be into the diaphragm. If this is not possible, weights could be too heavy.
- Don't let your shoulders creep up to your ears, i.e. keep your neck relaxed and your chin slightly tucked.
- Do gentle elbow extensions.
- You should feel your chest, shoulders and triceps working.
- Keep your weights over your chest, not over your eyes.
- Maintain your wrists in neutral or slight extension.

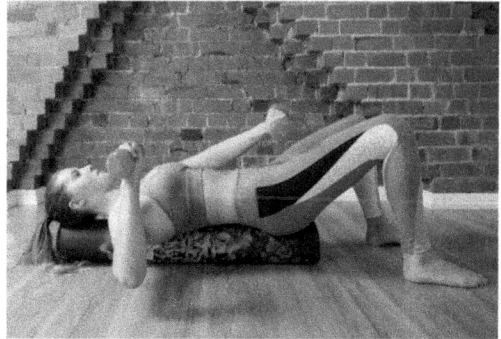

Make it harder:

- Include bench press as part of an upper body routine with triceps and flys.
- Do unilateral, across the body presses, *cross body pushes*. That is, push your right weight across your body over the top of the left hip and then return. Push your left weight across your body over the right hip and return. Either alternate your reps or do all reps in one direction and then repeated on the other arm.

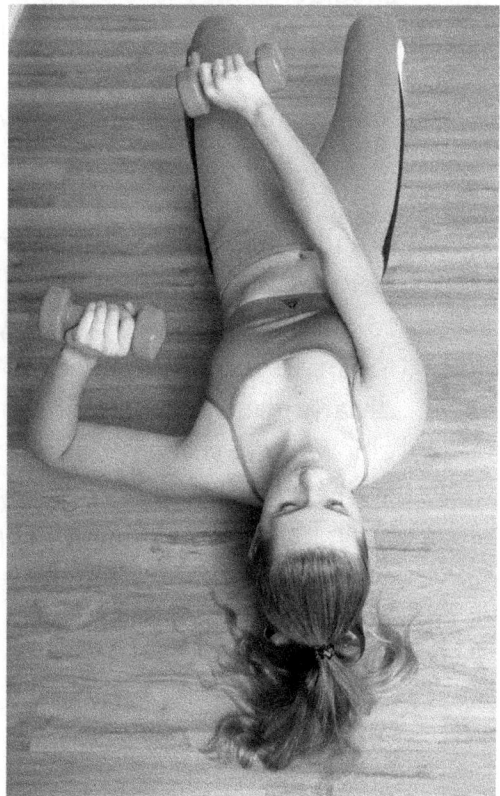

TRICEPS ON A ROLLER

Performing your tricep-strengthening on a roller gives you great feedback about your neck, shoulders and shoulder blade muscles positioning and activation. This is another great exercise to do as part of a neck rehab program as discussed above.

Set up:
- Supine lying on the roller, basic set up position.
- Weights in each hand, with your hands raised directly over each shoulder, with palms facing each other.
- Elbows are straight.
- Shoulder blade muscles are slightly engaged, i.e. squeezing a little around the roller.
- Keep your neck lengthened with chin slightly tucked.

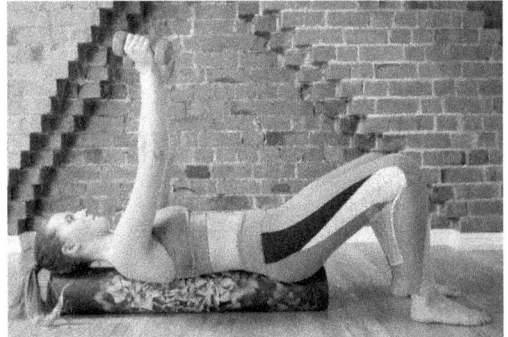

Steps:
1. Breathe in and slowly lower the weights by bending your elbow towards the outside of your forehead/top of the head.
2. Breathe out and straighten the elbows until you are back at your starting position.
3. Keep hands shoulder-width apart.
4. Try not to hit yourself in the head!
5. Repeat x10-15. 2-3 sets.

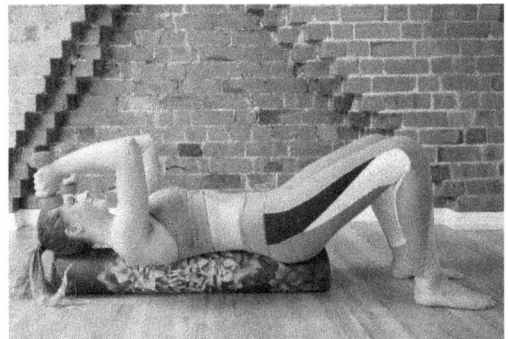

Tips:

- Try to keep the upper arms straight, i.e. perpendicular to your body and aligned with your shoulders. Your upper arms should not move out to the sides or down towards your chest while you are exercising.
- You should feel the back of your upper arms working, particularly as you get towards the end of the 2nd and the 3rd set, *if you are using the correct sized weight.*
- Keep your neck relaxed throughout the exercise. Your shoulders should not creep up to your ears.
- Maintain a neutral wrist position.

Make it harder:

- Perform alternating triceps extensions, i.e. right arm then left arm.
- Complete all the triceps extensions on one arm and then on the other.
- Include triceps as part of an upper body strengthening routine with bench press and flys. Perform 10-15 of each exercise with a starfish stretch in between each set. Do 2-3 sets.

FLYS ON A ROLLER

Flys is another upper body exercise that works shoulders, upper arms and chest. When you are performing unilateral flys on a roller you will be well aware of your core and its role in stabilising your body as you are using a weight at the end of a long lever. Sometimes it is necessary to decrease the size of your weights by 0.5-1kg if you are doing unilateral flys and find yourself compensating with knee movement or shoulder hitching.

Set up:
- Supine lying on a roller as per basic set up.
- Weights in each hand, your arms raised over your body, centred over your sternum.
- Your elbows are slightly bent, with your palms facing each other.
- Shoulder blade muscles are slightly contracted.

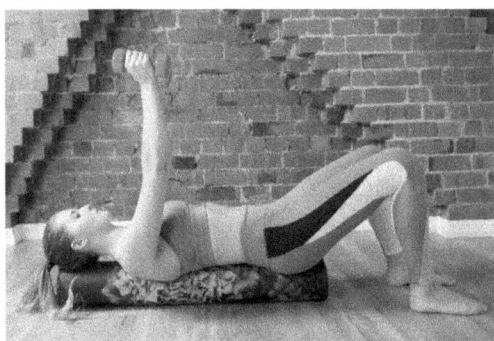

Steps:
- Breathe in and as you breathe out slowly lower your weights out to the side, until your arms are parallel with the floor.
- Breathe in and return slowly to your starting position, maintaining your slight elbow flexion.
- Repeat x10-15. 2-3 sets.

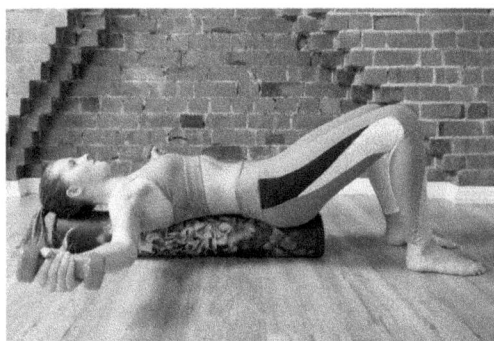

Tips:
- Keep your weights over your chest – do not let them creep up over your eyes.
- Don't pop your ribs, i.e. your thoracic spine should stay in contact with the roller.

Let it Roll

- Don't let your shoulders creep up to your ears, i.e. keep your neck relaxed and your chin slightly tucked.
- Maintain your wrist in a neutral or slight wrist extension position.
- Lumbar spine is neutral throughout.

Make it harder:
- Do unilateral flys, either alternating sides or doing all reps on one side then repeating all reps on the other side.
- Include flys as part of an upper body routine with bench press and triceps (as discussed).

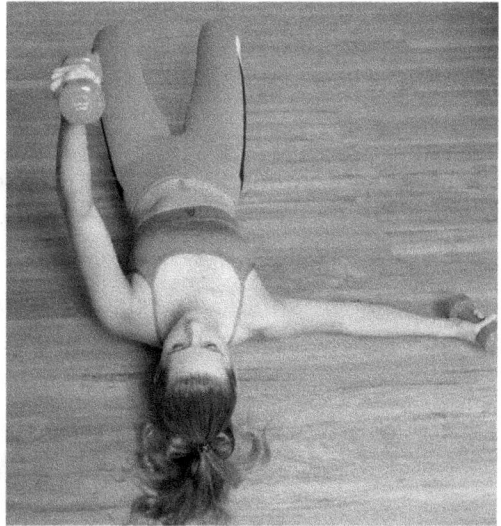

ROLLER 4-POINT KNEELING

4-point kneeling is a great core exercise that also works the deep stabilising muscles in the neck and at the shoulder blades. Adding in hip extension will work your glutes. With the roller 4-point kneel, we add an element of instability whether the roller is under the hands or beneath the knees. I have described both below. Try each version and see which one you prefer – they are harder than you think!

Set up A: Roller under hands
- Place your roller horizontally on the floor in front of you.
- Then, assume a 4-point kneeling position on the floor with your hands on top of the roller.
- Hands should *line up directly under your shoulders*. Your elbows should be straight but not hyperextended.
- If you were checking your side view in a mirror, your hips would be directly over your knees, and your pelvis and lumbar spine in a neutral position.
- Keep your neck lengthened, chin slightly tucked and eyes looking to the floor.
- Push your hands gently into the roller to turn on the shoulder blades muscles a little.
- Engage your deep tummy muscles gently as well.

Steps:
1. Take a breath in and as you breathe out raise your right arm out in front of your right shoulder. Pause. Then breathe in and return your hand to the roller. Make sure you turn on this right shoulder blade muscle again.
2. Breathe out and lift the left hand out in front of your left shoulder. Pause. Breathe in and return as above.

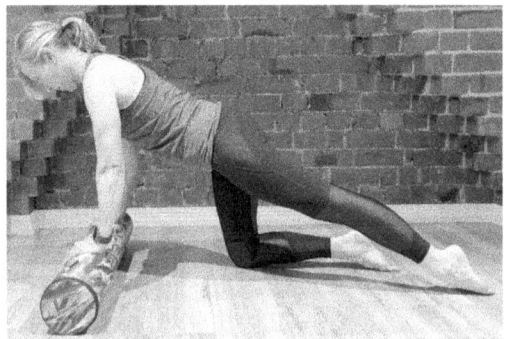

Let it Roll

3. Breathe out and slowly extend the right leg so that you straighten the knee in line with the right hip. Keep your big toe in contact with the floor. Pause. Breathe in and return the right knee to the floor, directly under the right hip.
4. Repeat with the left leg.
5. Continue until you have done 4-6 reps (each arm and each leg extension = 1 rep).

Tips:

- Maintain your neutral lumbar spine position throughout, especially as you swap from one leg to the other. You want to minimise any dropping or tilting of your pelvis.
- Initially, try not to lift your knee off the floor. Try to slide out your foot until your knee straightens and then slide back.
- Make sure knees remain hip-width apart; there is always a tendency to move them closer together.
- Try not to drop the head but ensure the neck is lengthened throughout.
- Knees should not hurt. Use a thick mat on the floor if they do.
- If your wrists are uncomfortable, try with the roller at your knees or attempt it using a half roller (semi-circular shape).

Make it harder:

- Slide your leg out and then lift your foot from the floor.
- Try extending the opposite leg with the outstretched arm (bird dog). Repeat x4-6 each side.

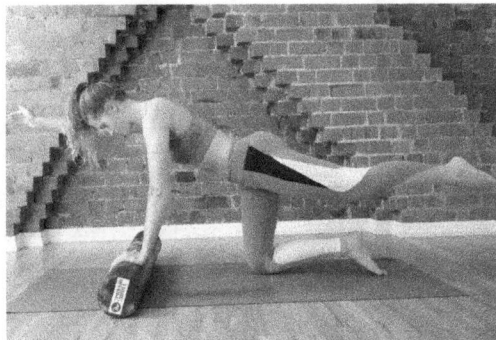

Set up B: Roller at knees

- Place your roller horizontally on the floor in front of you.
- Then, assume a 4-point kneeling position on the floor with knees (just below kneecaps) on top of the roller, with toes on the floor for support.
- Hands should *line up directly under your shoulders.* Elbows should be straight but not hyperextended or locked, knees under your hips.
- Neutral lumbar spine.
- Keep your neck lengthened, chin slightly tucked and eyes looking to the floor.

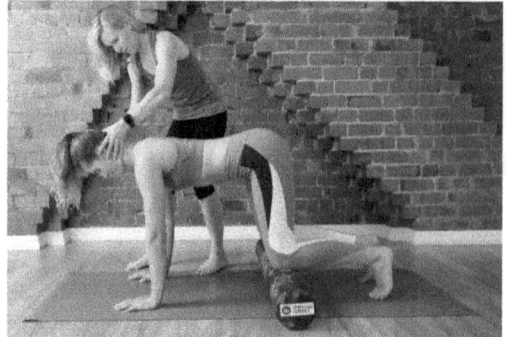

Steps:

1. Push hands gently into the floor to turn on the shoulder blades muscles a little.
2. Take a breath in and as you breathe out raise your right arm out in front of your right shoulder. Pause. Then breathe in and return your hand to the floor. Make sure you turn on this right shoulder blade muscle again.
3. Breathe out and lift the left hand out in front of your left shoulder. Pause. Breathe in and return as above.
4. Breathe out and slowly extend the right leg so that you straighten the knee. Keep your big toe in contact with the floor. Pause. Breathe in and return the right knee *slowly* to the roller. Slide it in directly under the right hip, so that there is minimal movement through the pelvis and spine.
5. Repeat with the left leg.
6. Continue until you have done 4-6 repetitions.

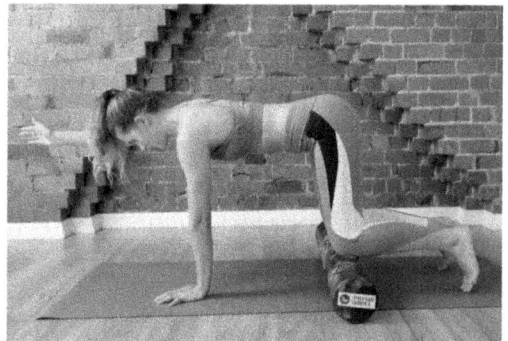

Tips:

- Maintain your neutral back position throughout to minimise any dropping of your pelvis.
- Keep your toes in contact with the floor. This will give you more stability. Try to slide out your toes until your knee straightens and then slide back.
- Make sure knees remain hip-width apart.
- Try not to drop the head but ensure that the neck is lengthened throughout.
- Knees should not hurt.
- If wrists are uncomfortable, use a small rolled up towel under the heel of your hands.
- You can also do just the arm lifts or just the leg extensions.

Make it harder:

- Slide the leg out and lift the foot to hip height then return.
- Slide the leg out and lift the opposite arm out. Repeat x3 each side.
- Lift the leg and opposite arm out and hold for 20-30 seconds. Return and repeat with the other arm and leg. See Bird dog page 132.
- Take both sets of toes off the floor to decrease your support and try all of the above variations.

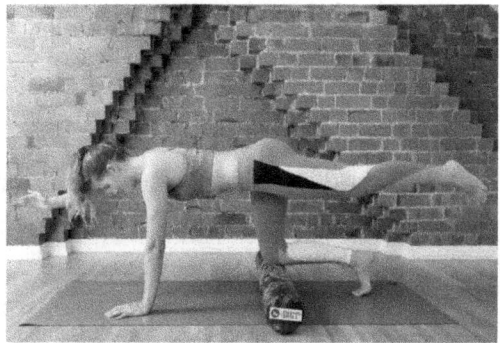

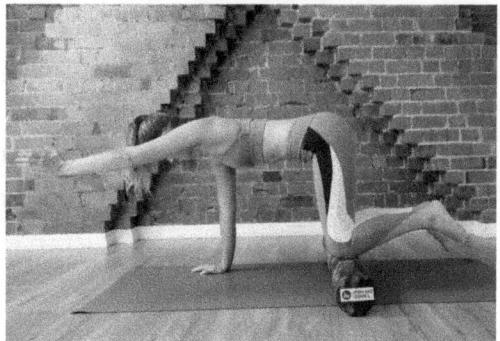

ROLLER PLANK ON KNEES

A plank is a demanding exercise that not only improves core strength but also works your shoulders, deep neck, glutes and quads. This is an intermediate version performed on your knees with the roller at your elbows. The roller adds instability and increases the height you have to lift and maintain your body at, above the floor.

Set up:
- Place the roller on the floor, horizontally.
- In kneeling, place the area just below your elbows on the roller, keeping your elbows directly under your shoulder joints.
- Keep your shoulder blade muscles gently contracted.
- Your chin should be tucked and your neck lengthened so that your head is in line with your body.

Steps:
1. Gently contract your deep tummy muscles.
2. As you breathe out, slide your knees back one at a time then lift and lengthen your torso so that ear, shoulder and hip joints are aligned.
3. Your lumbar spine should be in a neutral position.
4. Hold for 30-60 seconds, breathing normally into your diaphragm.

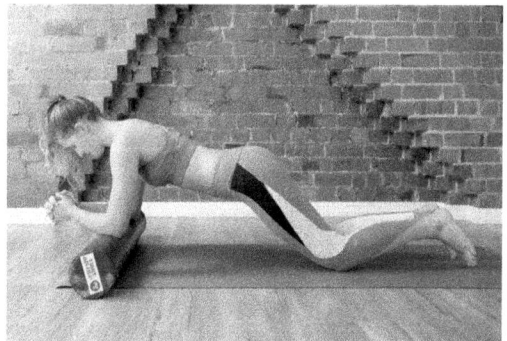

Let it Roll

Tips:

- If you experience back pain, **STOP**. You have fatigued your deep stabilising muscles and are now more than likely using your superficial back muscles, and they are not happy about holding this static position. The exercise is possibly too hard. Rest. Try again for a shorter length of time, say 15 seconds. Slowly add to the time you can hold it or try the plank on your knees without the roller.
- Don't drop your head or lift your hips out of alignment.
- Your shoulders and shoulder blade muscles need to be actively working.

Make it harder:

- Lift your knees off the floor and hold for 30-60 seconds (advanced plank - see page 140).

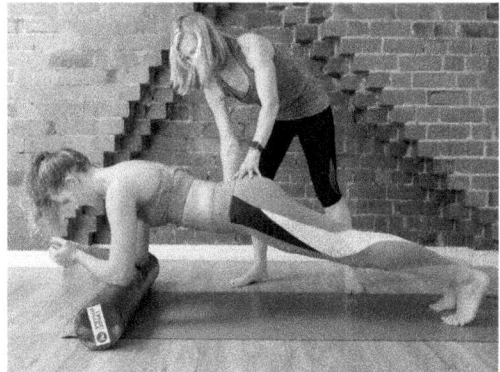

ROLLER PUSH-UP ON KNEES

Push-ups are a very common, functional strength training exercise that give a total body workout. This is a modified push-up on the knees. If you find it uncomfortable through your wrists try without the roller and then build up to adding the roller back in.

Set up:
- Place your roller on the floor, horizontally.
- In kneeling, place your hands on the roller, slightly wider than shoulder-width apart.
- Bring your shoulders over your hands, elbows will be bent.
- Keep your shoulder blade muscles gently contracted.
- Lengthen your body by sliding your knees back a little so that you are aligned through shoulders, hips and knees.
- Your lumbar spine is neutral.
- Your chin should be tucked and your neck lengthened so that your head is in line with your body.

Steps:
1. Inhale as you bend your elbows and lower your chest towards the roller, maintaining your body alignment.
2. Stop just short of the roller (or the range you can manage).
3. Then, exhale as you push through hands on the roller until your elbows are almost fully extended.
4. Repeat x10. 2-3 sets.

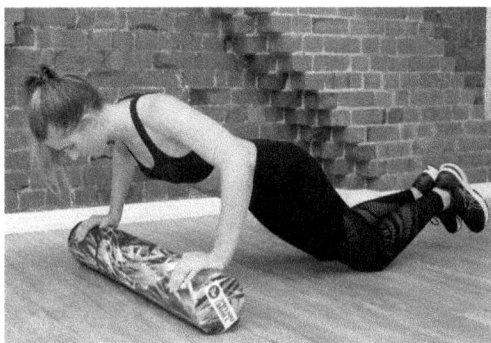

Tips:

- Don't let your head drop – focus on your chest lowering and maintain your alignment through ears, shoulders, hips, knees.
- Don't let your bottom stick up or lower back sag.
- There should be no neck or back pain.
- Thumbs should be next to fingers – don't stretch your thumbs around the roller.

Make it harder:

- Do a full push-up with the roller under your hands – see page 122.
- Try a full push-up with the roller at your feet – see page 123.

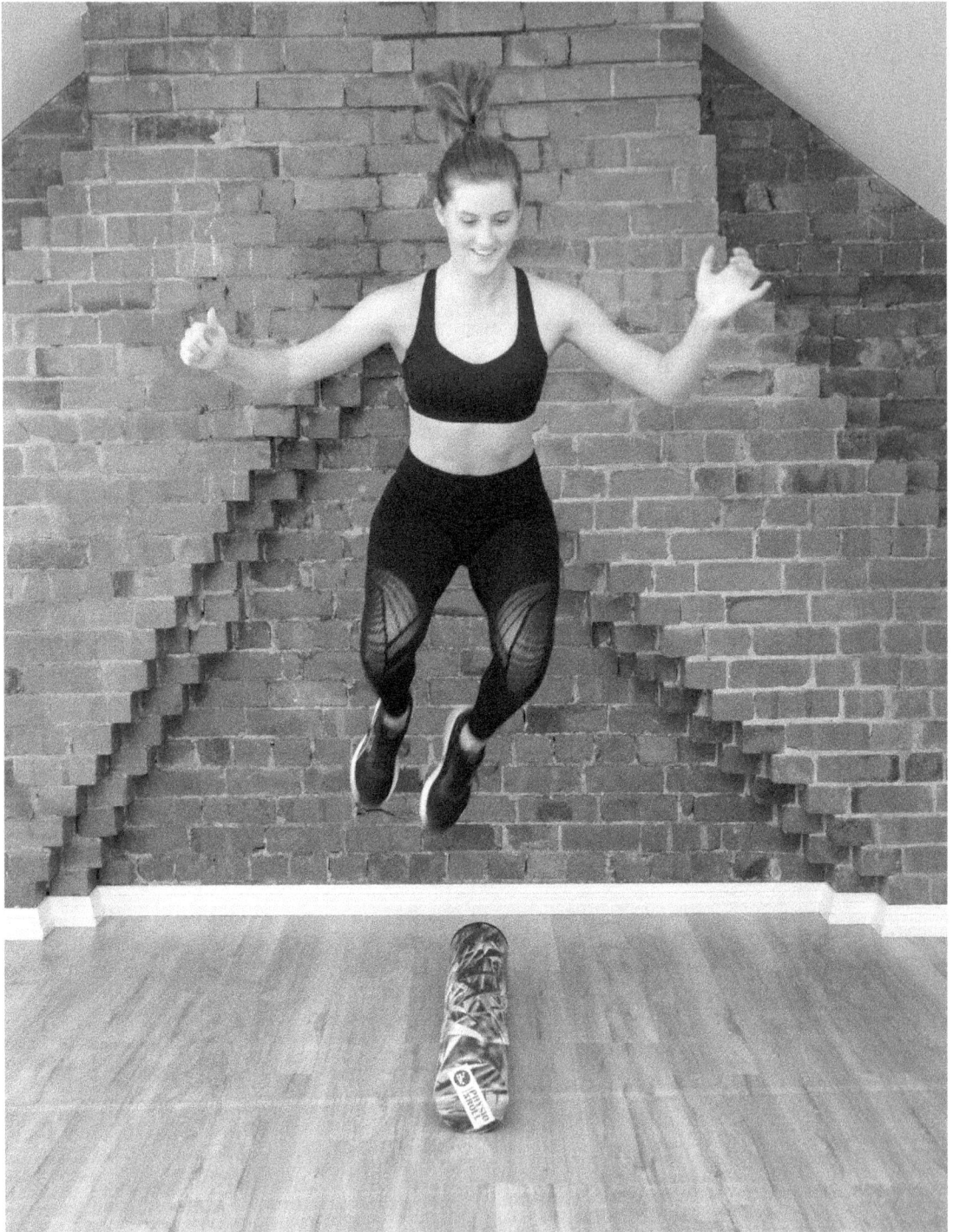

Let it Roll

CHAPTER 6

High Rollers

"Exercise not only changes your body, it changes your mind, your attitude and your mood."

Unknown

These are advanced exercises that build strength and control and add variety to your training. They are more complex than the exercises described in the previous chapters and should not be attempted if you are experiencing any back or neck pain.

PUSH-UP ON A ROLLER

Push-ups are a very common, functional strength training exercise that are a fast and effective way to boost upper body and core strength. Add in a roller, either at the feet or under the hands, to increase the difficulty. Try both versions and see which works better for you.

Doing push-ups every day can be effective if you are looking for a consistent exercise routine to follow. For best results continue to add variety to the types of push-ups you do. See "tips" for more variations.

Set up A: Roller under hands

- Place your roller on floor, horizontally/perpendicular to your body.
- Starting on your knees, lean forward and place your hands in line with your shoulders but slightly wider than shoulder-width apart, on the roller.
- Lengthen your legs and place your toes on the floor, hip-width apart.
- Gently tighten your deep tummy and shoulder blade muscles a little.
- Maintain your alignment through ears, shoulders, hips, knees and ankles.
- Tuck your chin slightly and lengthen neck, eyes looking to the floor.

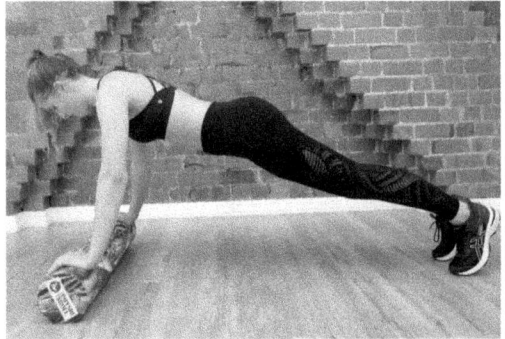

Steps:

1. Inhale as you bend your elbows and lower your chest towards the roller, maintaining your body alignment.
2. Stop just short of the roller (or the range you can manage).

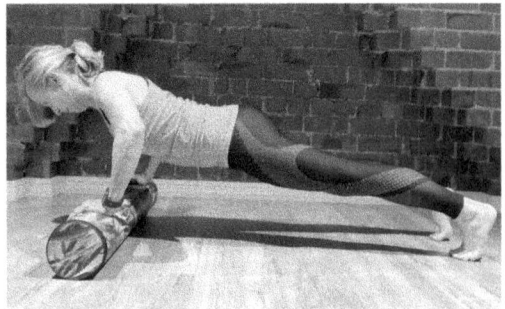

3. Then, exhale as you push through your hands on the roller till your elbows are almost fully extended.
4. Repeat x10. 2-3 sets.

Set up B: Roller at feet

- As above, have your roller on floor, horizontal/perpendicular to your body.
- Lay on the floor so that the front of each of your feet is on top of the roller, hip-width apart.
- Hands should be flat on the floor and positioned close to your shoulders.
- Gently tighten your deep tummy muscles and lift your body off the floor so your ears, shoulders, hips, knees and ankles are aligned.
- Draw your shoulder blades down and back, lengthen your neck and tuck your chin slightly – your eyes should look to the floor.

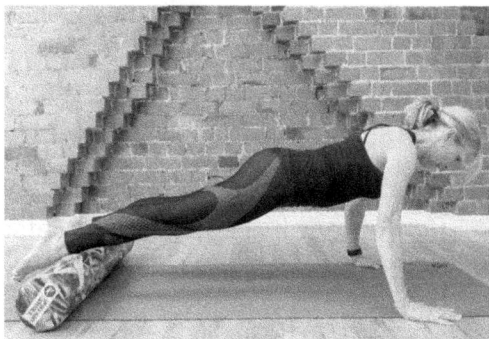

Steps:

1. Inhale as you bend your elbows and slowly lower your chest towards the floor.
2. Exhale as you push back up to your starting position.
3. Repeat x10+. 2-3 sets.

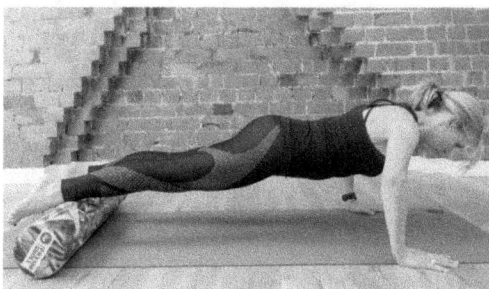

Tips:

- Don't let your head drop. Focus on your chest lowering and maintain your alignment through ears, shoulders, hips knees and ankles.
- Don't let your bottom stick up or lower back sag. Neutral lumbar spine.
- There should be no neck or back pain. Your shoulders and chest will be working hard.

Make it harder:

- Take one foot off the floor or roller and extend from the hip, holding while you do your reps x10. 2 sets.
- Do your push-up with your toes only on the roller x10. 2-3 sets.
- Perform mountain climbers (see page 130).
- Place the roller vertically under one hand and perform push-ups. Repeat x10 each arm. 2 sets.
- In this vertical position roll from one hand to the other as you perform your push-up. Repeat x10 each arm. 2 sets.

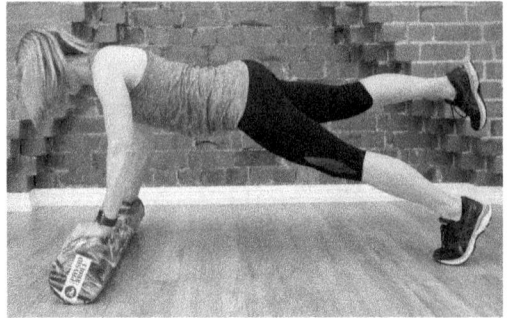

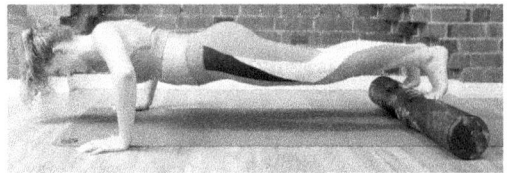

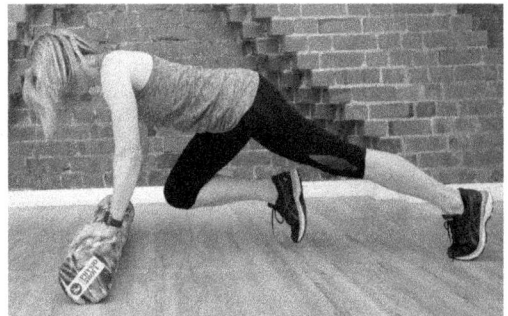

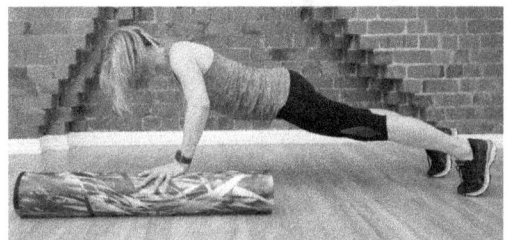

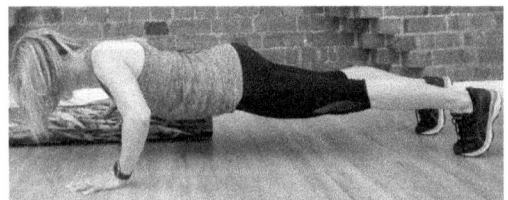

Let it Roll

ROLLER JUMPS

Roller jumps are a great addition to any exercise regime as they add a burst of cardio and help to build plyometric strength. Plyometrics refers to jump training; each time you land from a jump, your muscles get a stretch. That gives your next jump even more power. This combination of stretching and contracting your muscles boosts your muscle power, strength, balance and agility. You can either do a workout based around plyometrics or add a few plyometric-type moves to your usual routine.

Roller jumps is also great as an impact exercise to promote bone and cartilage health.

Set up:

- Place your roller on the floor/ground. Ensure you are on a stable, non-slip surface, with plenty of space around you and preferably with sneakers on.
- Stand beside your roller, side-on, about halfway along its length.
- Feet should be about hip-width apart.

Steps:

1. Bend your knees and hips and jump sideways with both feet over the roller, landing with knees and hips slightly bent.
2. Bend your knees and hips and jump back.
3. Repeat x20-30. 2-3 sets.

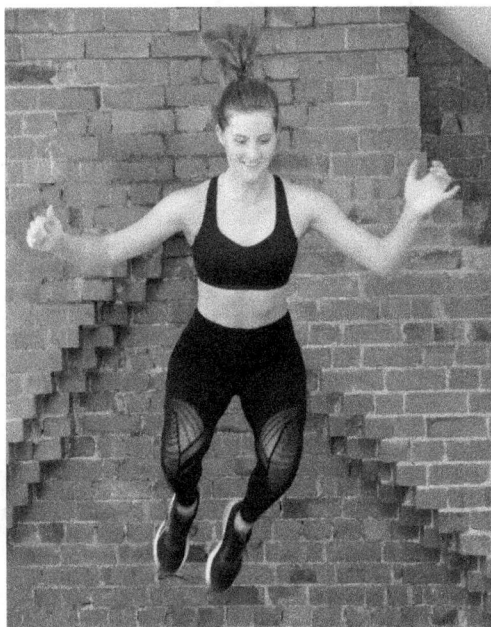

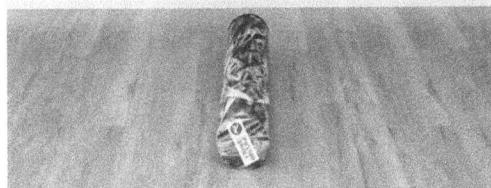

Tips:
- Try to land evenly, with feet flat and knees soft.
- If you accidentally touch your roller, stop and make sure it has stopped moving before you start jumping again.
- Use your arms for momentum, to increase your roller jump height and for balance.
- Mix double feet jumps with single leg hops.

Make it harder:
- Turn to face your roller and jump forwards over it, then jump backwards.
- Try not to pause after each jump, making your jumping continuous.
- Repeat x20-30. 2-3 sets.

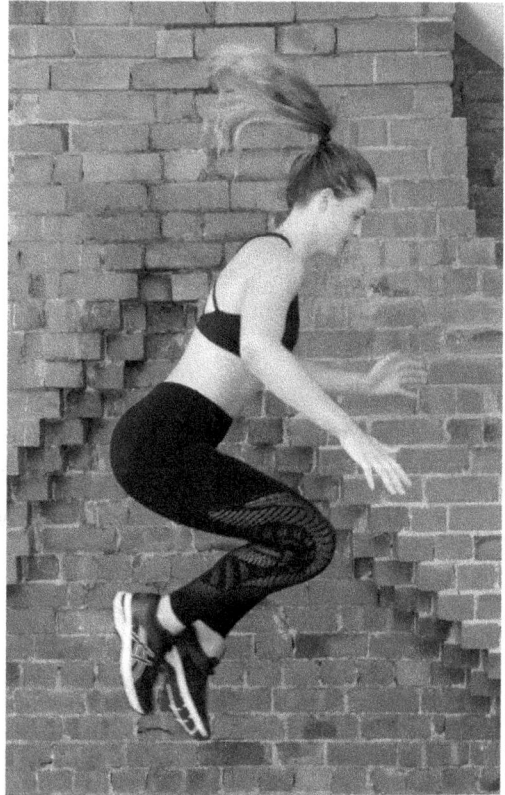

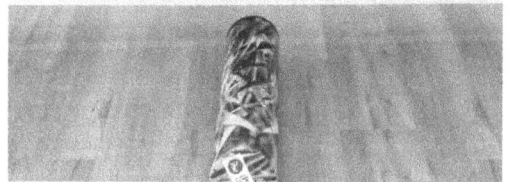

ROLLER LUNGES

Lunges are a lower body unilateral exercise that challenge your quads, glutes, core and balance. This version with a roller can be tricky to set up initially but can be varied to suit your skill level (see tips). Add hand-weights or a band to increase the complexity and also strengthen your upper body. You can perform this exercise with or without shoes.

Set up:

- In standing, feet hip-width apart, place your roller horizontally behind you on the floor so that it is in contact with both heels (or shoes).
- Take a large step forward with your *left* foot.
- Maintaining pressure into your *left* heel, lean forward slightly from the hips to help place the toes and ball of your *right* foot on top of the roller (NB. You may want to stand beside something for support when you first attempt this. Alternatively, place the roller against a wall to minimise its movement when first starting the exercise if you are unstable).
- Then re-align your ear, shoulder and hip over the back knee.
- Lumbar spine is neutral.
- Both feet should still be hip-width apart.

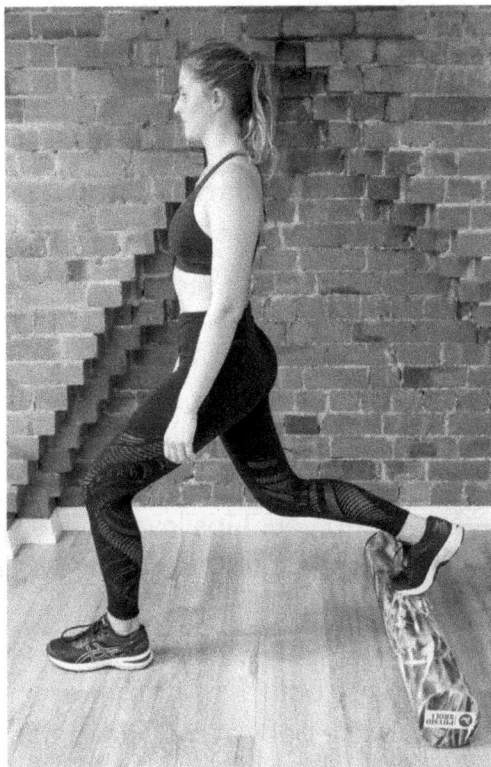

Steps:

1. Keep pressure into your *left* (front) heel and inhale as you slowly lower the *right* knee directly down towards floor.
2. Try to keep your left knee from moving beyond your *left* big toe.
3. Exhale as you push through the heel and straighten the front knee back to your starting position.
4. Repeat x15-20.
5. You should feel your glutes working hard on your *left* (front) leg and your quads working as hard (or harder) on the *right* (rear) leg.
6. Swap to your right foot on the roller and repeat x15-20. 2-3 sets.

Tips:

- Ideally, stand in front or side-on to a mirror so that you can check your alignment throughout the exercise.
- Your rear knee should point directly to the floor, not move medially or laterally.
- The front kneecap should stay in line with your 2nd toe.
- Keep weight into the front heel throughout the roller lunge to activate your glutes.
- Try to have the front shin aligned vertically, i.e. front knee over front ankle.
- Keep your hips level.
- There should be no knee pain.

Make it harder:

- Raise both arms straight out in front of the body at shoulder height and maintain while performing your lunges, as shown. Alternatively, hold the arms out to the sides in line with shoulders.
- Add hand-weights and do bicep curls, lateral raises, overhead press or scaption unilaterally or bilaterally.

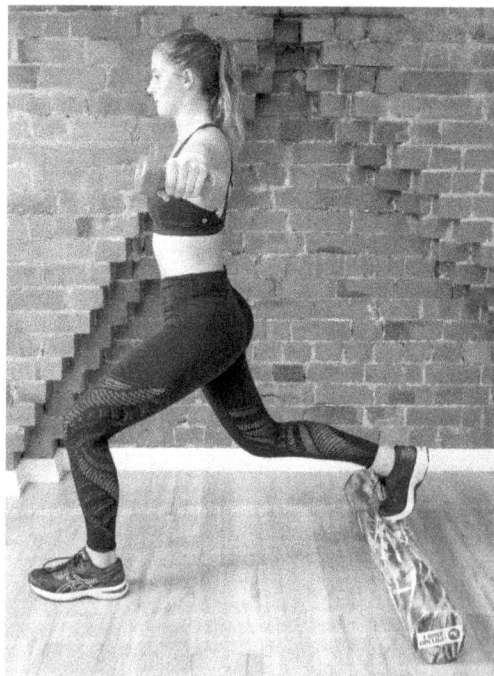

Let it Roll

- Add a resistance band beneath the ball of the front foot and perform bicep curls, lateral raises or scaption bilaterally or unilaterally as you lower the back knee.
- Lunge as above but hold in the low point of the lunge and then move roller back and forth x10 before returning to the starting position and repeat x15-20.

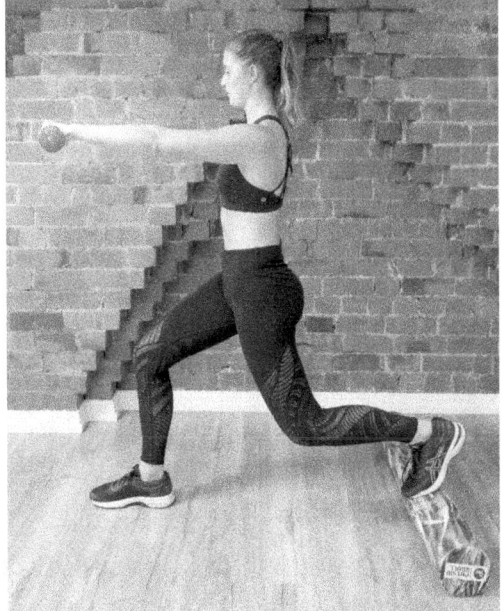

MOUNTAIN CLIMBER

Performing a mountain climber with a roller is an advanced abdominal exercise that is great for scapula (shoulder blade) stability as well as shoulder and core strength.

Set up:
- Place your roller horizontally/perpendicular to the body, on the floor.
- Assume a push-up position on the roller, i.e. your hands on the roller (thumb next to the fingers), slightly wider than shoulder-width apart but aligned under your shoulders, legs straight, toes on the floor, hip-width apart.
- Gently tighten your deep tummy and shoulder blade muscles. Neutral lumbar spine.
- Ears should align with your shoulders, hips, knees and ankles.
- Chin slightly tucked, neck lengthened, your eyes looking to the floor.

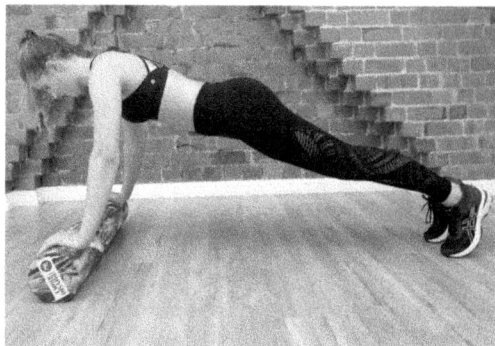

Steps:
1. Inhale and bend your left knee and bring the knee in a straight line towards the chest.
2. Exhale and return the left knee to starting position.
3. Inhale and bend right knee and move it towards the chest.
4. Exhale and return the right knee to your starting position.
5. Repeat x10-20 each leg, alternating sides. 2-3 sets.

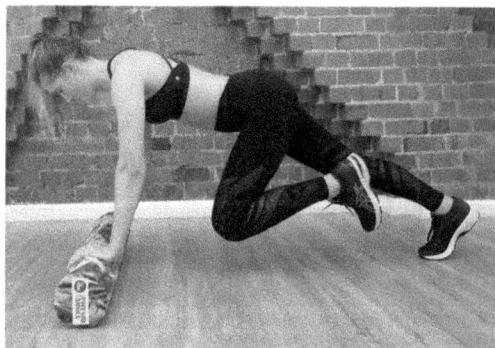

Tips:

- Make sure your feet stay hip-width apart throughout to help with your stability.
- Don't switch on your neck muscles, keep your neck lengthened, chin tucked and shoulder blade muscles engaged throughout.
- Maintain your neutral lumbar spine and hip/shoulder alignment.

Make it harder:

- Bend your left knee and move it diagonally towards the right shoulder then return. Move your right knee towards your left shoulder. Repeat x10-20.

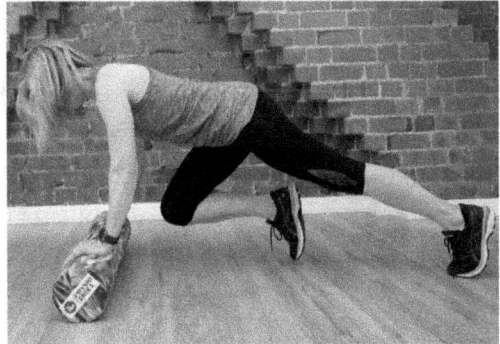

- Perform the knee flexion towards the chest on the left leg only x10-20 repetitions and then repeat on the right.
- Increase the repetitions to x30 each leg.
- Perform a combination of push-up and mountain climbers; e.g. x10 push-up then x10 mountain climbers, alternating each leg.
- Put the roller at the shins, hands on floor and stabilise through upper body. Perform the mountain climber either rolling both knees towards the chest or bringing a single knee towards the chest as the other leg stays extended. There are videos of these harder options on the *Physio on a Roll* website.

BIRD DOG ON A ROLLER

Add in a foam roller to a basic bird dog and the deep stabilising muscles in the torso, neck and scapula are further challenged. There are many variations to this exercise. I have described one option below; see the "make it harder" section for alternatives.

Set up:

- Place your roller horizontally on the floor, in front of you.
- Then, lower your knees *hip-width apart*, so that you are kneeling on top of the roller. The area of your knee just below your kneecap should be in contact with the roller. Your toes should still be touching the floor.
- Move your hands to the floor in front of you. They should *line up directly under your shoulders*, elbows straight but *not hyper-extended, elbow creases facing in*.
- If you were checking your side-view in a mirror, your hips would be directly over your knees, and your pelvis and lumbar spine would be neutral.
- Keep your neck lengthened, chin slightly tucked and eyes looking to the floor.
- Push gently into the floor with your hands and turn on your shoulder blade muscles.

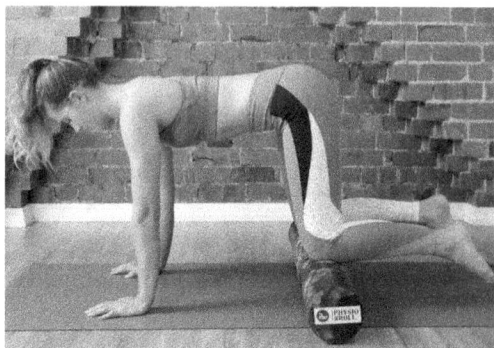

Steps:

1. Take a breath in and as you breathe out raise your right arm out in front to shoulder height, while simultaneously extending your left knee out behind your body, to hip height.

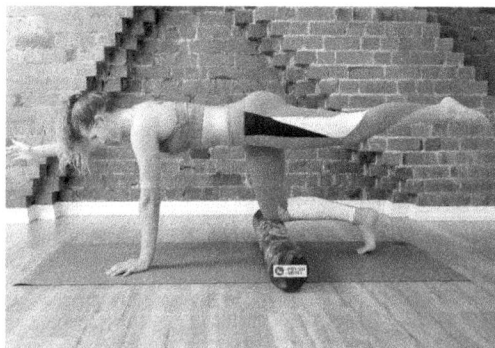

2. Maintain your neutral lumbar spine and left shoulder blade contraction.
3. Breathe in and return your arm and leg to their starting positions, re-engaging your right shoulder muscle.
4. Breathe out and repeat with your left arm and right leg.
5. Perform x10 each side. 2-3 sets.

Tips:
-   Try to do bird dog side-on to a mirror to check on your alignment initially and then by turning your head during the exercise.
-   Try not to lift knee off the roller – instead slide the leg out. This will help to maintain your neutral lumbar spine.
-   Don't drop your head; keep chin tucked and neck lengthened.
-   Your knees should not hurt.

Make it harder:
-   Lift the toes from the floor on the supporting leg.
-   Hold in the extended position for 10 seconds before returning to the start position and swapping to the other side.
-   Roll the roller down to the front of the ankles. Maintain hip and knee flexion at 90° and perform arm and leg extension as above.

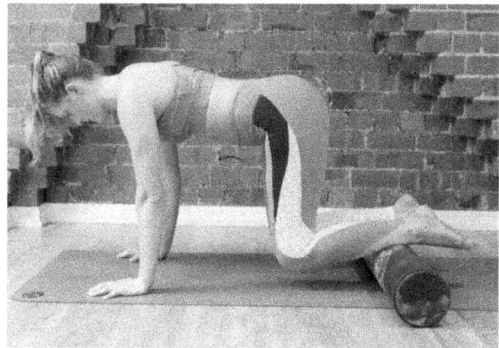

ADVANCED ROLLER BRIDGE

If you have mastered a basic roller bridge then this is a great progression. By placing the roller under your feet, you increase your instability. You have to really focus to ensure that you maintain your glute contraction and pelvis alignment.

Set up:

- Supine on the floor with your feet on the roller, positioned in the middle 1/3 of the roller as shown. Your roller should be perpendicular to your body and within a foot's length of your bottom.
- Feet and knees are hip-width apart and you can have shoes on or be barefoot.
- Try to have your heels and/or the area a little towards your mid-foot, on the roller.
- Arms should be relaxed by your sides with palms facing up towards the ceiling and shoulders rolled down and back towards the floor. Relax your neck.

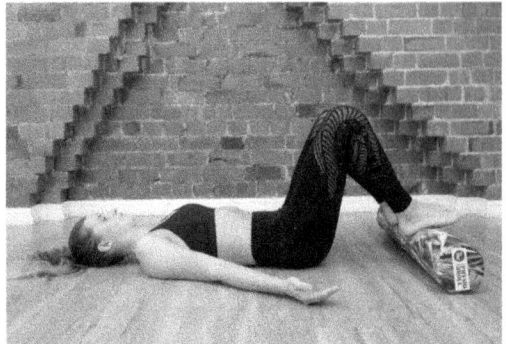

Steps:

1. Breathe out, tilt your pelvis (to flatten your lumbar spine into the floor) then squeeze your bottom muscles.
2. Then push through your heels on the roller to slowly lift your pelvis, one vertebra at a time, off the floor. Lift until your knees, hips and shoulders are aligned. Lumbar spine is neutral.
3. *Maintain downward pressure through your heels onto the roller.*

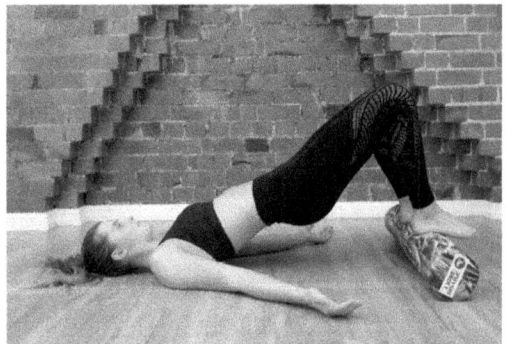

4. Breathe in and lower one vertebra at a time towards the floor, until your tailbone touches the floor.
5. Repeat x10. 2-3 sets.

Tips:

- Make sure that you *maintain downward pressure through your heels onto the roller.* If you push out, the roller, as it is a cylindrical shape, will roll out and away and you will feel your hamstrings, at the back of your thighs, contract, often uncomfortably!
- Try not to overarch your lumbar spine or lift your pelvis too high.
- You want to feel your bottom working, not your hamstring muscles.
- There should be no knee pain. Move your roller slightly away from your bottom to use your quads less and ease knee discomfort.
- Relax your neck and shoulders and keep your shoulders away from your ears even though you will weight-bear through your upper back and shoulders.
- There should be no back pain. Reassess your positioning and ensure that you are using your bottom muscles. If back pain persists, try the basic bridge on a roller and its harder options.

Make it harder:

- Once in your advanced roller bridge, lift the right foot off the roller, straighten the right knee (so that it lines up with the right hip) and hold for 3-5 seconds. Make sure you keep your pelvis level. Then lower the right foot back to the roller and lower your bottom back to the floor. Repeat on the left.

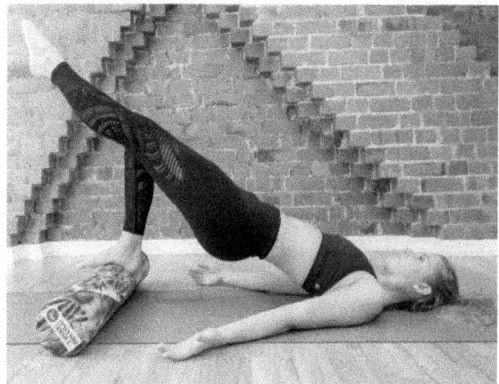

- Add a resistance band around the tops of your knees and move either both knees or a single knee in a bent knee fall out.
- Add a weight over your pelvis as you lift (Gus the pug in this case!).
- Head to the *Physio on a Roll* website for more variations.

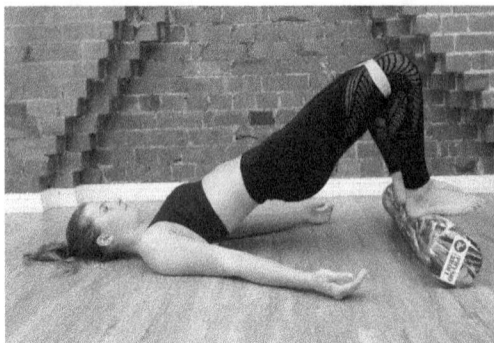

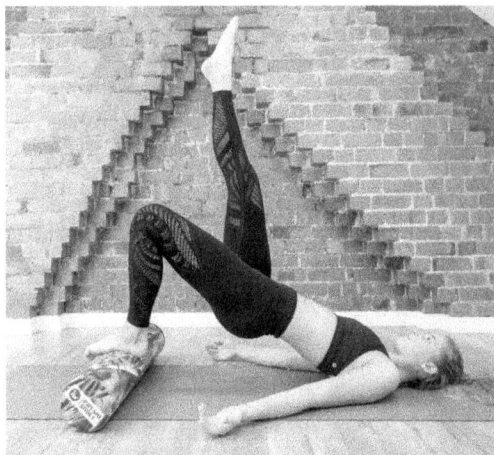

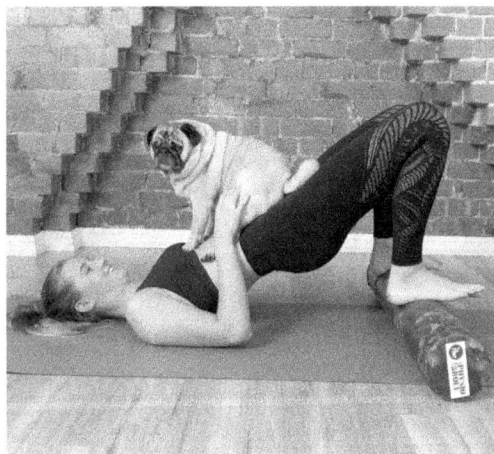

Let it Roll

DRINKING BIRD

Drinking bird (single leg deadlift) is a hip-hinge movement that strengthens the back, core and legs. It is a great exercise for advanced balance training because the entire sequence requires you to stand on one leg while extending the other leg behind you.

Watch the video of this exercise on the *Physio on a Roll* website for clarity.

Set up:
- Standing on one leg, knee slightly bent.
- Other leg extended from the hip behind body, knee straight.
- Lumbar spine is neutral.
- Hands on each end of the roller, arms raised overhead, elbows straight.

Steps:
1. Keep weight into the standing heel as you bend forward *from the hips* for the first third of the movement (a "hip hinge").
2. Continue to bend through your knee, hips and lumbar spine to take the roller towards the floor but try not to touch the floor.
3. Return slowly to the upright starting position, keeping weight into the heel, your knee slightly bent and your arms straight while holding the roller.
4. Repeat x10.
5. You should feel your glutes (where your back pocket would sit) on the standing leg working++.
6. Change legs and repeat x10. 2-3 sets.

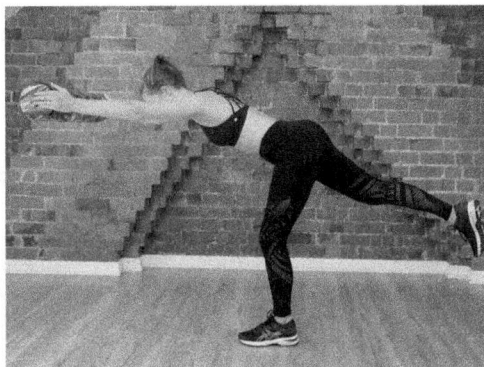

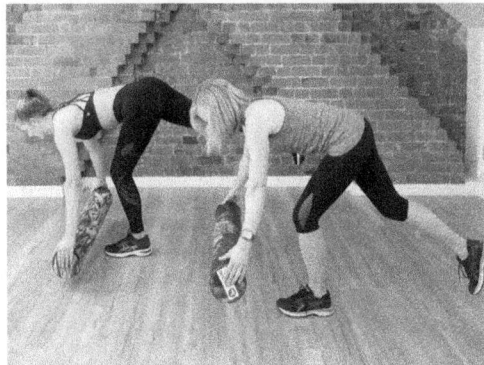

Tips:

- Try to keep your weight into your heel, especially as you return from the lowered position, to help maintain your balance.
- Keep the elevated leg extended throughout exercise to help with balance.
- Try to keep pelvis facing forward without rotating, twisting or hitching one hip.
- Your head should stay within your arms until your arms go towards the floor.

Make it harder:

- Move the outstretched leg to in front of the hip, bending the knee, as you simultaneously lift the roller up from the floor position to the overhead position. Repeat x10. 2-3 sets.

Let it Roll

PLANK ON A ROLLER

A plank challenges the entire body and boosts core strength. When you add a roller, either at the shins, toes or elbows, you add an unstable base to your performance, amplifying the difficulty.

Set up A: Roller at ankles

- Lay face down on the floor.
- Place your roller on the floor perpendicular to your body, adjacent to the ankles.
- Feet and knees are hip-width apart, but your knees and hips are resting on the floor.
- Your forearms and hands are also resting on the floor, with the elbows directly under the shoulders.

Steps:

1. Inhale, then exhale and gently contract your deep tummy and shoulder blade muscles, push into your arms and lift your body off the floor, so that ears align with shoulders, hip, knee and ankle joints.
2. Lumbar spine is neutral.
3. Your chin should be slightly tucked and your head in line with your body, eyes gazing at the floor at fingertip level.
4. Keep breathing normally into the diaphragm.
5. Maintain your deep tummy contraction and squeeze your bottom muscles.
6. Hold for 60+ seconds.

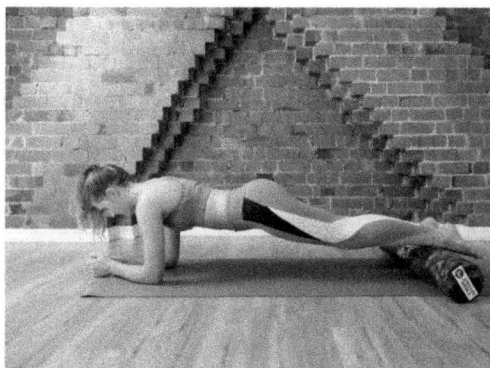

Set up B: Roller at elbows
- Place your roller on the floor, horizontally.
- In kneeling, place your upper forearms (close to the elbows) on the roller. Keep the elbows directly under the shoulders.
- Switch on your shoulder blade muscles and lengthen your torso.
- Your knees and feet are resting on the floor.

Steps:

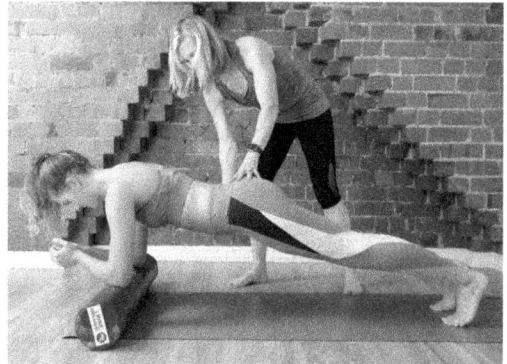

1. Inhale, then exhale and gently contract deep tummy and shoulder blade muscles, push into forearms and lift your torso from the floor so that your ear, shoulder, hip, knee and ankle joints are aligned.
2. Lumbar spine is neutral.
3. Continue to breathe normally into your diaphragm.
4. Your chin should be slightly tucked and your head in line with your body.
5. Hold this position for 60+ seconds.

Tips:
- Don't let your bottom lift towards the ceiling or your tummy sag towards the floor.
- Try not to let your head drop towards the floor.
- Your shoulders and shoulder blades will be working hard.
- If you experience back pain, **STOP**. Your deep muscles have fatigued and now you are fatiguing the surface back muscles. Rest. Try again for a shorter duration. Or move the roller to the forearms. If you are still having difficulty try the plank with your knees on the floor (intermediate plank) for a longer duration.
- A phone with a counter placed within sight helps enormously with this exercise.

Make it harder:

- Lift one leg into extension and hold for 30 seconds, then repeat with the other leg, again holding for 30 seconds. Make sure you maintain your alignment throughout.
- Try the roller underneath your hands (similar to a push-up starting position).
- Move the roller so that only the toes are on top of the roller and repeat as above.

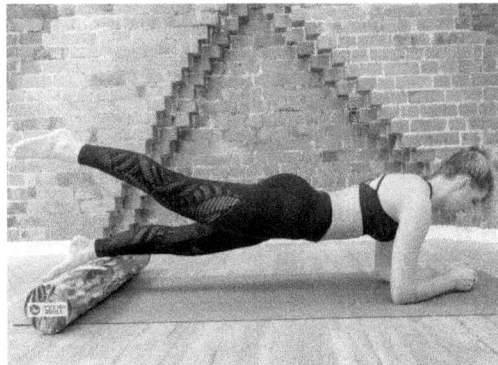

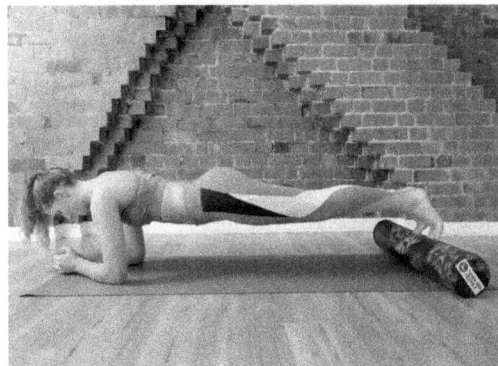

SIDE PLANK ON A ROLLER

Side planks are another great core exercise that particularly target your quadratus lumborum muscle in your lumbar spine and your obliques. Use a mat or carpeted floor to help cushion the forearm and prevent slipping. It is harder than it looks!

Set up:
- Side lying on the floor with the roller placed perpendicular to the body, at ankle level.
- Place your feet so that heel of one foot touches the toes of the other foot.
- Your forearm is on the floor, parallel to the roller, with your elbow located directly under the shoulder joint.
- Your ear should be in line with your shoulder joint, your hip joint and where your feet meet on the roller.

Steps:
1. Inhale, then as you exhale tighten your deep tummy and shoulder blade muscles, push into your forearm using your shoulder and lift your hips from the floor so that your nose aligns with your sternum and belly button.
2. Raise your upper arm vertically over your shoulder.
3. Keep your lumbar spine neutral.
4. Maintain your lower shoulder blade contraction and squeeze your buttock muscles.
5. Breathe normally and hold for 30-60 seconds.
6. Lower slowly to the floor, repeat on the other side.

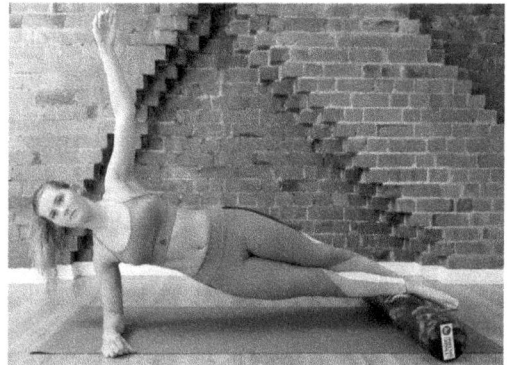

Tips:
- Make sure your pelvis does not rotate anteriorly or posteriorly.
- If you experience shoulder or neck pain, stop, lower to the floor, and

reposition your elbow beneath the shoulder joint. Then engage the shoulder blade muscles and start again. If you are still feeling pain, use your free hand to squeeze your shoulder joint.

- Similarly, if you experience back pain, stop, check your hip/pelvis alignment and start again or limit to 10-20 second holds. If you still feel back pain, stop and go to an easier front plank version (on the knees) of this exercise before trialing this exercise again.

Make it harder:
- Place one ankle on top of the other (instead of the straddle position described above).
- Lift the top leg, keeping the knee straight, and hold for 30-60 seconds.
- Have your hand on the floor (directly beneath your shoulder, elbow straight) instead of your forearm and repeat the exercise as described above.

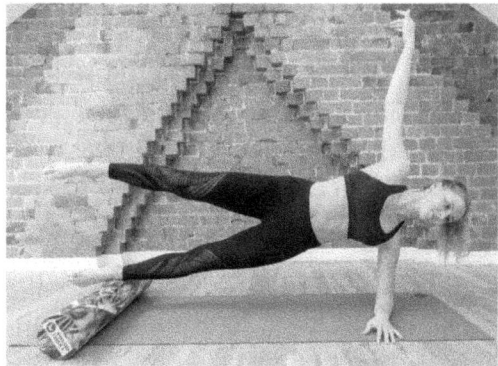

ADVANCED ABDOMINALS – TOE TAPS

This is a little more challenging than the single then double leg lift. Be aware of your lower back positioning throughout.

Set up:
- Supine on the roller in basic set up position.

Steps:
1. Inhale, and as you exhale slowly lift the right knee above the right hip.
2. Inhale, then exhale and slowly lift the left knee above the left hip.
3. Inhale and slowly lower your right foot to "tap" the toes on the floor, then exhale and return so that the right knee is again over the right hip.
4. Inhale and slowly lower the left foot towards the floor, "tap" the toes, then exhale and return so that the left knee is again over the left hip.
5. Repeat x5-10 each side. 2-3 sets.

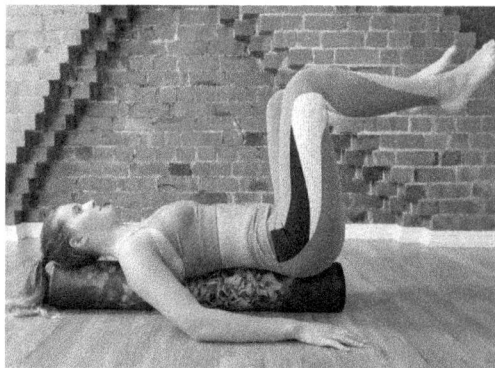

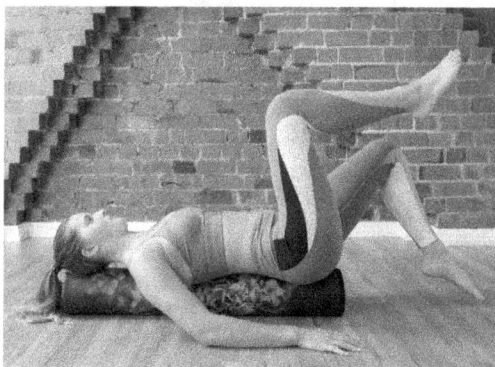

Tips:
- The lower back will move a little closer to the roller with both knees positioned above the hips. Take care not to *arch* the back or *"squash"* it into the roller.
- You should not feel the lower back pulling or feel pain.
- Similarly, the neck should not pull or hurt.
- Don't let the ribcage *"pop"*.
- Try not to hold your breath.

- If you cannot perform the exercise without these compensations then go back to the easier option of *single then double knee in the "Now You're on a Roll' chapter.*

Make it harder:
- Progress to elbow support only on the floor.
- Repeat the toe tap on one side only first, then the other.
- Increase the repetitions to x20.

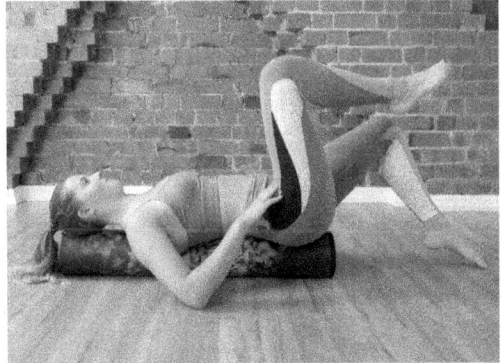

ADVANCED ABDOMINALS – SINGLE LEG EXTENSION

Set up:
- Supine on the roller in basic set up position.
- Both forearms should be resting on floor beside roller.

Steps:

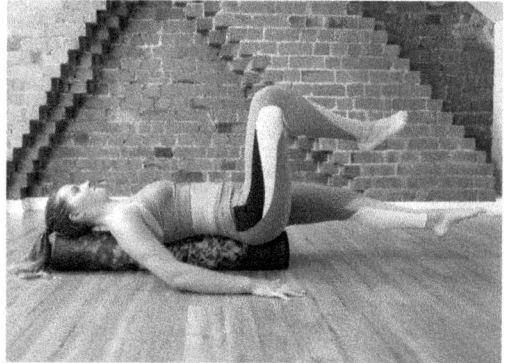

1. Inhale, then exhale and slowly lift right knee so that it sits directly above right hip, then lift left knee directly over left hip.
2. Exhale as you slowly straighten the right knee, lowering the leg until it is parallel with the floor.
3. Inhale as you bend the right knee and return it to above the right hip.
4. Repeat with the left leg.
5. Repeat x5-10 each leg.
6. Then slowly lower right foot to the floor and then left foot to the floor.
7. Repeat 2-3 sets.

Tips:
- Do not hold your breath, or arch or squash your lumbar spine into the roller.
- You should not experience back pain/neck pain or pulling. If you do, stop. Try the toe taps exercise which is slightly easier with knees bent. You could also do less repetitions or not lower your extended leg as far.
- Keep your neck and shoulders relaxed throughout.

Make it harder:
- Take your forearms off the floor and just use elbow support.
- Do up to 20 repetitions (each leg).
- Try a bicycle on a roller (see the Physio on a Roll website for instructions).

ROLLER BETWEEN KNEES

This exercise is another advanced abdominals exercise.

Set up:
- Supine on the floor with knees bent, feet and knees hip-width apart.
- Neutral lumbar spine.
- Roller beside you on the floor.

Steps:
1. Inhale, then exhale and slowly lift right knee above right hip.
2. Repeat with the left knee over the left hip.
3. Reach for the roller and position it between your knees and feet.
4. You will need to squeeze a little with feet and knees to stop it falling. There should be roller sticking out past your feet and past your knees.
5. Inhale and as you exhale move knees, roller and feet to the right (around 1 o'clock), inhale and return.
6. Exhale and move to the left, inhale and return.
7. Continue to alternate sides.
8. Repeat x10 each side.
9. Then lower legs slowly to the floor.
10. Repeat (2 sets).

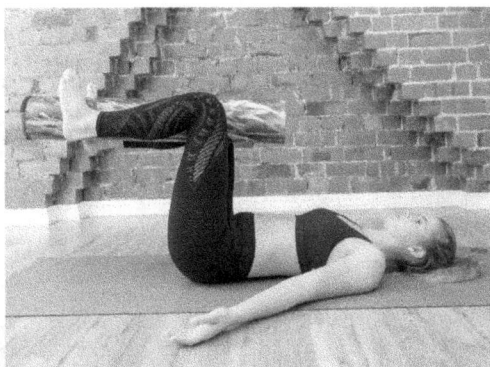

Tips:
- Don't arch or squash your lumbar spine into the floor; it will be close to the floor but just maintain that position.
- Don't let your body rock from side to side. Just do small range movements.
- Keep your knees directly over your hips.

- There should be no back pain. Decrease your reps or go back to an easier abdominal exercise if your lumbar spine is uncomfortable.

Make it harder:
- Push the roller that is between the knees until it is flush with the knee joints and it sticks out past the feet. Breathe in and as you breathe out lower the knees, the feet and the roller towards the floor to touch the end of the roller on the floor. Breathe in and return slowly. Don't hold your breath, let your back arch or squash into the floor. Repeat up to x10. 2 sets.

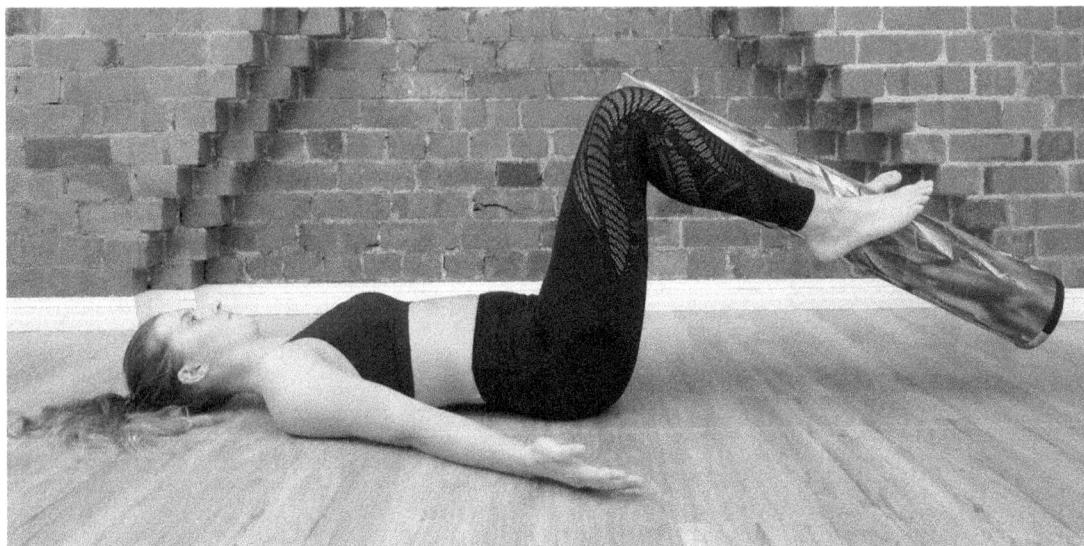

TRICEPS DIPS ON A ROLLER

Triceps dips on a roller are an advanced body-weight exercise. The triceps muscles are underneath your upper arm and help to straighten both the elbow and shoulder joints. Performing a triceps dip on a roller requires core and shoulder blade activation to stabilise you as you lower your body towards the floor using your triceps muscles.

Set up:

- With your roller on the floor, sit on the floor with your bottom and lower back adjacent to the middle of the roller (as in the photo).
- Knees are bent and your feet and knees are hip-width apart.
- Reach your hands behind you onto the roller and position the hands with fingers facing forward, directly beneath your shoulders.

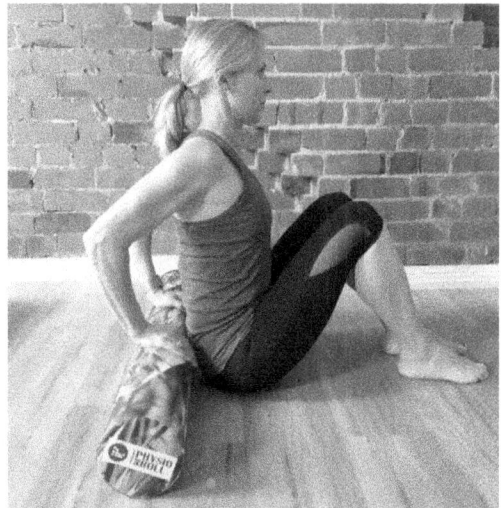

Steps:

1. Inhale and gently draw your shoulder blades down and back.
2. Exhale, push down on the roller and straighten your arms so that you lift your bottom off the floor.
3. Keep your elbows pointing directly behind you, and your forearms perpendicular to the floor.
4. Then inhale and slowly bend your elbows to lower your body straight down towards the floor. Keep your bottom close to the roller, but don't touch the floor.

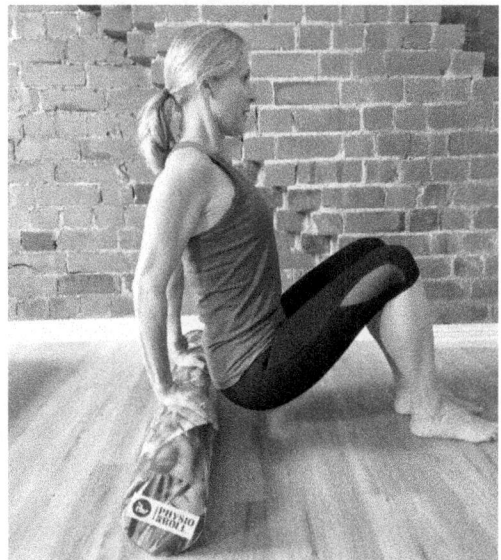

5. Exhale and push down on the roller as you straighten your elbows and return.
6. Repeat x10-15. 2-3 sets.

Tips:
- Make sure that you keep your shoulders away from your ears, with your neck relaxed.
- Maintain your shoulder blade contraction to keep your chest open.
- Your head/ear should be in line with your body.
- Keep your elbows pointing behind you throughout the triceps dip.
- Try not to touch the floor with your bottom.

Make it harder:
- Straighten your knees so that your legs and feet are hip-width apart in front of you. Your heels are resting on the floor. Then follow steps 1-6 as above.
- Keep your legs straight and place one foot on top of the other, crossing at the ankle. Then continue your triceps dips as above.

CHAPTER 7

Roll and Release

"Be not afraid of going slowly, be afraid of standing still."

Chinese proverb

The following exercises are a comprehensive guide to mobilising your body, using either a foam roller or heavy resistance band. Many of the roller massages may be familiar but do follow the tips for alignment to get the best out of each exercise.

ROLLER REACH AND SQUEEZE

Roller reach and squeeze is essentially a shoulder blade exercise, but it also benefits the thoracic spine, neck and shoulders. The repeated protraction/retraction actions train the stabiliser muscles around the shoulder blades. And, because of the shape and positioning of the roller, the thoracic spine and neck receive a great mobilising effect.

Set up:
- Supine lying on the roller, basic set up position.

Steps:
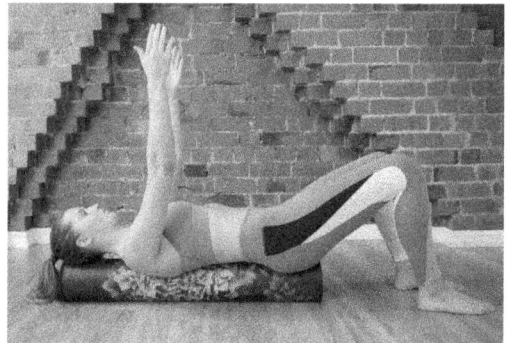
1. Raise both arms in the air so that your hands are directly over your shoulders, palms facing each other.
2. Gently squeeze both shoulder blades together around the roller.
3. Then gently reach both hands a little towards the ceiling, using your shoulder blade muscles only.
4. Repeat x10.
5. Then repeat x5-10 each arm on its own.

Tips:
- Keep your upper neck muscles relaxed. If you reach too far these muscles will activate.
- Keep your elbows straight.
- Remember to breathe normally throughout the roller reach and squeeze exercise.
- Try not to "pop" your ribs, i.e. your upper back should stay relaxed.

Make it harder:

- Add in circles bilaterally and unilaterally.
- Add in scissors or shoulder range of motion exercises.

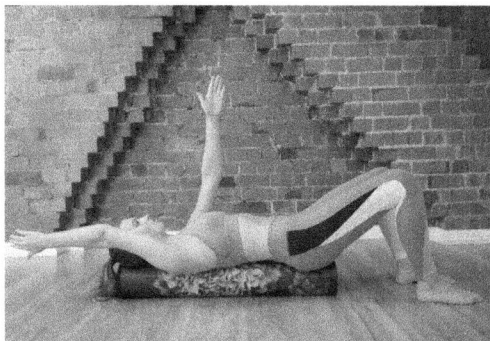

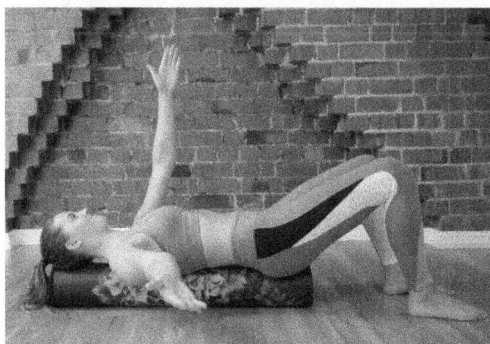

STARFISH STRETCH

The starfish stretch is a simple, feel good stretch that helps to reverse the *sitting, head forward posture* that many of us assume when working at a desk, day in, day out. It stretches the chest, pecs and shoulders, hip flexors, cervical, thoracic and lumbar spine and ribs.

Set up:
- Supine on the roller, basic set up position.

Steps:
1. Slowly move your arms out from the body to approximately the 10 o'clock and 2 o'clock positions, if you think of the analogy of a clock face.
2. Slowly stretch your legs out to approximately 4 o'clock and 8 o'clock.
3. Your lumbar spine will flatten towards the roller.
4. Breathe normally into the diaphragm.
5. Maintain this position for 30 second or longer.

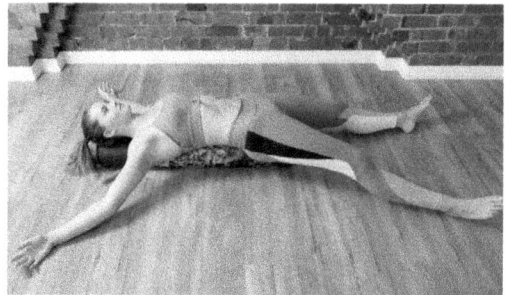

Tips:
- You should feel a moderately strong but not uncomfortable stretch at the shoulders/chest/pecs area.
- If it is uncomfortable, move your arm(s) a little to find a more tolerable position.

Make it harder:
- Bend your elbows and, keeping them close to the floor, move both your arms slowly up in a semi–circle till they meet above your head and then slowly return – this is known as snow angels.

HIP FLEXOR STRETCH

Your hip flexors are also known as iliopsoas. They are a strong muscle group that originates from the front of your lumbar vertebrae and extends to your femur/ thigh bone. They can feel tight if you sit for prolonged periods.

Set up:

- In supine lying, knees bent, feet and knees hip width apart.

- Place your roller horizontally under your thighs, close to your buttocks, with both palms placed at the ends of the roller.

Steps:

1. By pressing your heels into the floor, lift your buttocks off the floor (into a bridging position) and move the roller with your hands so that the roller rests under the sacrum, i.e. above the coccyx, but below the lumbar spine (as pictured right).

2. Gently draw your left knee towards the chest, using your hands around the back of the left thigh to increase the stretch.

3. Lengthen the right leg along the floor, trying to straighten the right knee as much as possible. You should feel a moderately strong stretch at the top of the right thigh/in front of the right hip. Hold for 20-30 seconds.

4. Bend the right knee so that right foot is again flat on the floor. Lower the left foot back to the floor.

5. Repeat with your right knee into the chest as per the steps above.

Tips:
- There should be no back pain or discomfort.
- The roller should feel comfortable under the sacrum – if not, reposition.
- The stretch at the front of the hip should only be mild to moderate. Do not try to increase the stretch or hold for too long.

THORACIC ROLL OUT

Thoracic roll out on a roller mobilises the thoracic spine and is useful for easing neck pain and neck stiffness. It can be varied to suit your desired level of massage. Initially it can be quite uncomfortable, especially if you are particularly tight or stiff around your neck to mid back area. Persevere if you can, doing frequent rolls of short duration, as it does make a difference to your neck and thoracic mobility with time and practice.

Set up:
- In supine lying, with knees bent and feet hip width apart.
- Place your roller, perpendicular to the spine, underneath your shoulder blade area.
- Place your hands behind your head, keeping your elbows in line with your ears.

Steps:
1. Keeping weight into both of your heels, squeeze your buttocks and lift your pelvis off the floor, so that your hips line up with your shoulders and your ears.

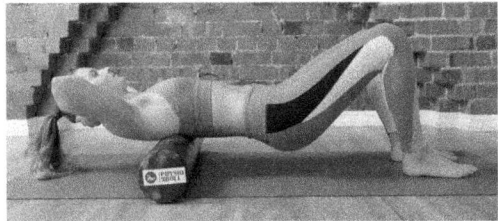

2. Use your heels to move your body back and forth over the roller and over the shoulder blade area only.
3. Continue for 40-60 seconds.

Tips:
- Breathe normally throughout the exercise.
- Maintain a neutral lumbar spine.
- Keep your chin slightly tucked and your elbows in line with your ears throughout the exercise.
- Squeeze your bottom muscles and maintain this contraction throughout the exercise.

THORACIC EXTENSION ON A ROLLER

This is a great mid back mobility exercise which also helps with neck or shoulder pain and tightness. It works well with the thoracic roll out exercise, especially if that is performed first.

Set up

- Sit on the floor with your hips and knees bent and feet flat on the floor.
- Put the roller about 40cm behind you, on the floor, perpendicular to your body.
- Lay back on the roller so that it sits at the base of your shoulder blades.
- Then put your hands behind your head, interlacing your fingers and keeping your elbows pointing forward.

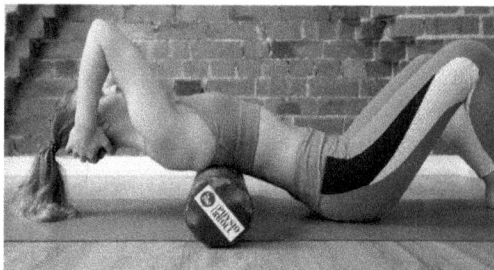

Steps:

1. Take a breath in and as you breathe out, slowly lower your upper body towards the floor, over the roller.
2. Your hands should be supporting your head.
3. Just move in the range that is comfortable.
4. Return to the starting position and then slide your buttocks a little further along the floor away from the roller, so that the roller is now positioned around one vertebra higher on your thoracic spine.
5. Breathe in and again, as you slowly breathe out, lower your upper body towards the floor.
6. Repeat another 2 times through, so that you have done 4 reps.

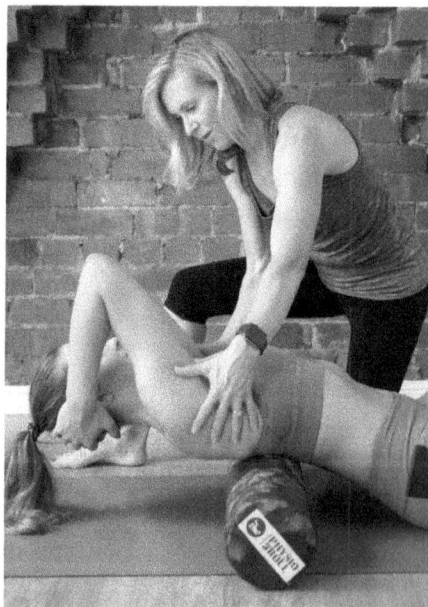

Tips:

- Thoracic extension with a roller can be quite an intense exercise. If it is too uncomfortable, stop. Go to thoracic roll out instead.
- You may hear a pop or click – this is okay. It is just a joint self-manipulation.
- Make sure you support your neck with your hands throughout the thoracic extension movement.
- Don't hold your breath.

WINDMILL STRETCH

Windmill stretch uses breathing and repeated movements to gently restore rotation to the thoracic spine. Lack of mobility in the thoracic spine can be associated with neck and shoulder pain. This exercise also stretches your pectoral muscles.

Set up:
- In side-lying, knees on top of each other and bent to 90°, positioned directly in front of your hips.
- Ear, shoulder and hips aligned.
- A pillow (or two) under your head for support, so that your neck is in a neutral position, i.e. aligned horizontally with the thoracic spine.
- Your arms are stretched out in front of your shoulders or lower arm can be bent as shown above.
- The roller is parallel to the body and under the palm of the outstretched upper hand.

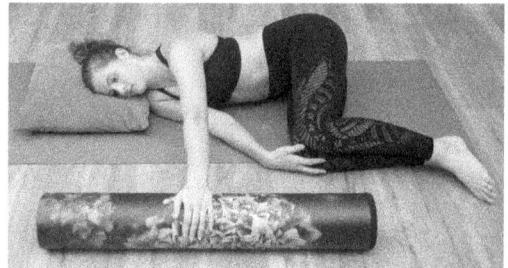

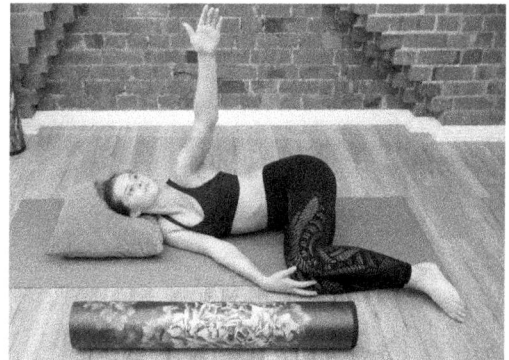

Steps:
1. Breathe in and gently reach forward by using your shoulder blade (protraction), rolling the roller forward a little.
2. Breathe out and retract back, again by using the shoulder blade and then, keeping your elbow straight, lift your hand off the roller and sweep the arm up and over to reach behind the body, palm facing upwards.

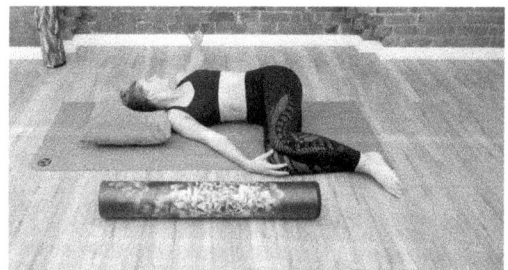

3. You are trying to get the back of your hand to the floor, or if your hand can touch the floor easily, try to get the upper shoulder blade near the floor.
4. Breathe in and bring the arm back up and over, keeping the hand in line with shoulder.
5. Repeat the same process x6-10.
6. With the last repetition, hold the outstretched position behind the body and breathe in deeply, then breathe out deeply and move your hand, arm and shoulder blade slightly further into range.
7. Repeat on the other side x6-10.

Tips:

- Your head can follow your hand movement or it can stay facing forward; choose what is comfortable.
- Try not to let the top knee move from the bottom knee – keep them squeezed together.
- You should do normal breaths into the diaphragm throughout; adding a deep breath at the end of your repetitions, to improve your range.
- If the stretch at the pecs is too strong or uncomfortable, bend the elbow as it leaves the roller and keep the palm of the hand close to the body, near the ribcage, and try to move only the upper shoulder blade closer to the floor with each repetition (known as a bow and arrow movement).

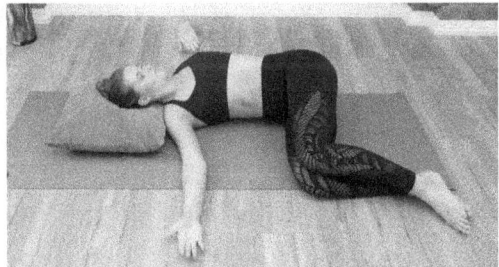

QUADS MASSAGE WITH A ROLLER

This massage is for the powerful muscles that sit on the front of the thigh; the quadriceps. It can be quite uncomfortable but does improve with practice. Try to roll the entire length of your quads initially to see where you are most uncomfortable and then concentrate on that area. Be sure to keep your toes on the floor if you find that the quads release/massage is really unpleasant.

Set up:
- Place the roller on the floor, perpendicular to your body.
- Gently lower your body to the floor so that the front of the thighs, about mid-thigh level, are resting on the roller.
- Your forearms should be resting on the floor, elbows aligned under your shoulders, with knees and toes resting on the floor.
- Your chin should be lightly tucked with your neck lengthened and your ears aligned with your shoulders, hips and ankles. Neutral lumbar spine.

Steps:
1. Gently contract your shoulder blade muscles and then lift knees and toes from the floor. Keep your legs straight and hip-width apart.

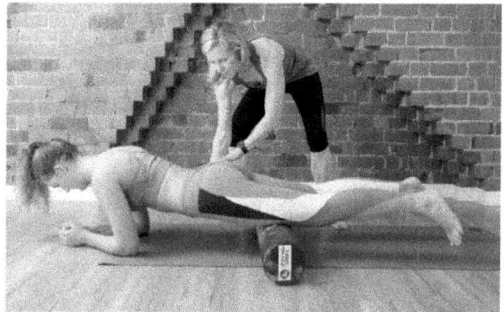

2. Using your forearms, gently roll along the length of your thigh or quads muscles, from hip level to knee level.
3. Continue for 1-3 minutes, concentrating on particularly "tight" areas, going back and forth either side of the tight area, as tolerated.

Tips:

- If it is too uncomfortable, keep your toes on the floor. If it is still difficult to tolerate, take more body weight through your forearms.
- Try to keep your chin tucked and your head in line with your body throughout with your neck and shoulders relaxed.
- Don't let your back sag – maintain your lumbar spine in neutral.
- You should also try the ITB release if you find this quads massage beneficial. These two releases work well together.

ITB MASSAGE WITH A ROLLER

The ITB (Iliotibial band) is a thick fibrous band of fascia that originates from the Tensor Fascia Lata (TFL) and glute max muscles. It travels over the hip and inserts just below the knee. The ITB is often involved with hip and knee issues and rolling it out can have positive effects on knee and hip pain and mobility.

ITB massage with a **roller** is a common exercise but is often poorly performed, with little thought given to the rest of the body's positioning during the exercise. The description below emphasises head and body alignment and use of your core muscles and shoulder blade for stability. Placing your foot flat on the floor in front of your body also allows you to vary the amount of weight that you lower onto the roller. This set up means that if you find the ITB release *really uncomfortable* (which it can be!) you can use your forearm and foot to lift some of your body weight off the roller.

Set up:

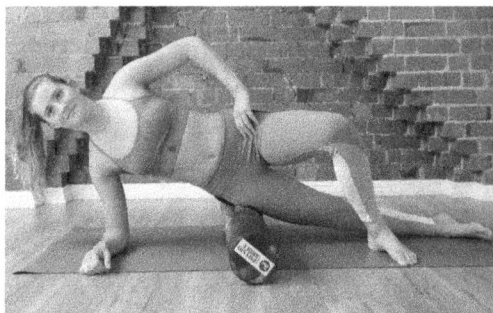

- Roller on the floor, so that it will be horizontal/perpendicular to the body.
- Position yourself side-on to the roller so that your right hip/outside of the right upper thigh is on the roller.
- Keep the right knee straight and the outside of the right foot resting on the floor.
- The right forearm should be flat on the floor with your right elbow directly underneath your right shoulder, with your right shoulder blade muscles switched on a little.
- Align your right shoulder with the right hip, right knee and right ankle (the side you are massaging).
- Your left leg should have the knee and hip bent. Then place your left foot flat on the floor, in front of your body, to support your body weight on the roller.

Steps:

1. Lift the foot of the leg being massaged off the floor.
2. Maintaining your alignment, use the arm on the floor for momentum and roll the outside of the leg along the roller.
3. Find the areas of discomfort and massage back and forth over them.
4. Continue for 2-3 minutes as tolerated.
5. Repeat on the other leg.

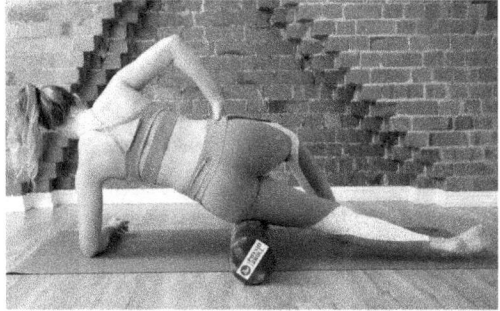

Tips:

- Concentrate on the areas that are tight or "gnarly" – this may be anywhere along the ITB, at your hip or near your kneecap.
- If this is too uncomfortable, take more body weight through your forearm, or the foot that's on the floor in front. Maybe leave the outside of the foot on the floor (of the leg you are massaging) or roll for 30-40 seconds only.
- It will feel better with repeated sessions over several days.

Make it harder:

- Change the plane of the movement so that at the hip, for example, the pelvis tilts slightly to massage the ITB closer to the insertion into the glute.
- Lift the foot off the floor in front and place this leg on top of the other. This will add to the weight on the roller.

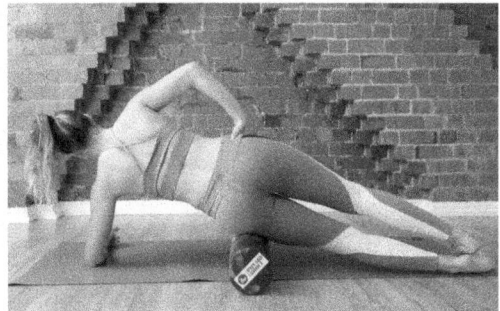

LEG STRETCHES (HAMSTRING, GLUTES, ITB, ADDUCTORS)

This series of leg stretches are for the **hamstrings**, **glutes**, **ITB** and **adductors** or inner thigh muscles. They are presented together as it is simple to go from one stretch to the next, safely and effectively. The set up described is designed to minimise any strain on the neck, shoulders and lumbar spine. These are best performed with a heavy resistance band or with a towel. Watch the full sequence via the video on the Physio on a Roll website.

Set up:

- Supine lying on the floor, with or without a pillow underneath the head as needed.
- Loop a heavy resistance band around the ball of the left foot, holding an end in each hand.
- Raise the left leg toward the ceiling, maintaining a little bend at the knee.
- Pull on the ends of the band so that the resistance in the band holds the weight of the leg, then rest the elbows on the floor, beside the body.
- The elbows and the band should be holding the weight of the leg.
- Your neck and shoulders are also relaxed.
- Lumbar spine in a neutral position.
- Breathe normally.

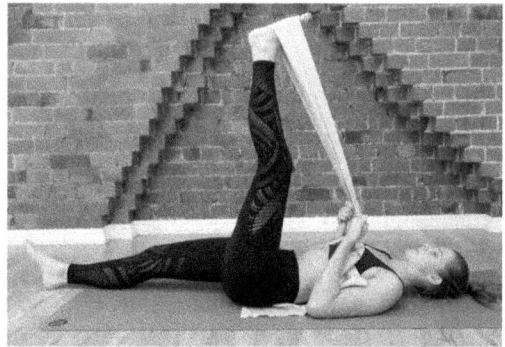

Steps:

1. Bend the left knee slightly and move it towards the chest a little so that you feel the stretch only in the back of the thigh (**hamstrings stretch**) and not behind the knee. Hold for 20-30 seconds, breathing normally throughout.
2. Gently point your toes towards the ceiling and then back towards your body to add in a **sciatic nerve mobilisation**. Repeat x15-20.

Let it Roll

3. Then swap both ends of the band into the right hand.

4. Lower the left leg, straightening the left knee as you lower and draw the leg over the right side of the body, to feel a stretch on the outside of the left hip (**ITB stretch**). Often you need to lengthen the torso on the left-hand side or stretch your left hip towards the right foot which is on the floor. Ensure that the elbow and the band are still holding the weight of the leg and that you are not hitching your hip on the left or lifting your back too far from the floor.

5. Hold for 20-30 seconds, breathing normally throughout.

6. Then bend the left knee and draw the left knee and left foot in with the band towards the right shoulder; you should feel a stretch in your left buttocks (**glutes stretch**).

7. Hold for 20-30 seconds, breathing normally throughout.

8. Then swap both ends of the band back to the left hand, and with the left elbow on the floor beside the body, holding the weight of the leg, slowly swing the left leg out to the left side, in the range that is comfortable, so that you get a left inner thigh stretch or groin stretch (**adductor stretch**).

9. If this last stretch is too strong or uncomfortable in your lower back, bend the right knee and put the right foot on the floor.

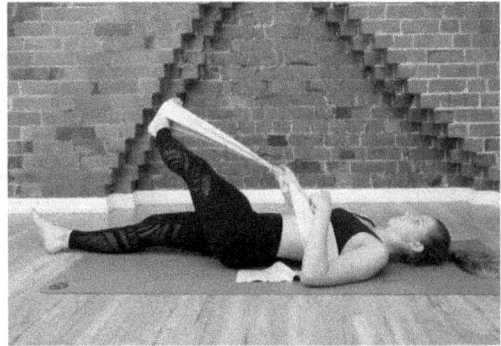

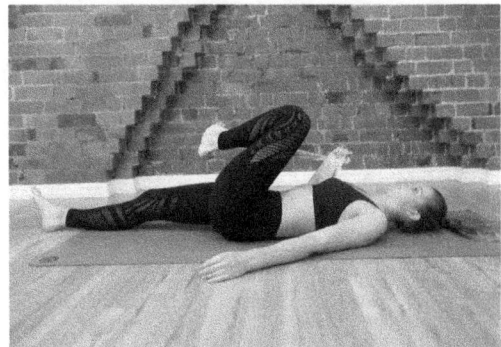

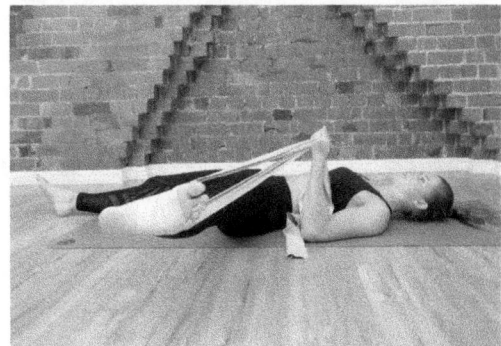

10. Hold the stretch for 20-30 seconds, breathing normally throughout.
11. Repeat the above sequence on the right leg.

Tips:

- You should not feel back pain whilst performing the stretches. If you do, bend the knee of the leg you are not stretching and place the foot flat on the floor.
- You are after a moderate to moderately strong stretch only; the stretch should not be uncomfortable.
- Make sure neck and shoulders stay relaxed throughout.

QUADS STRETCH IN STANDING

This is a simple, fast and effective stretch, for the muscles at the front of the thigh.

Set up:
- In standing, lumbar spine neutral, feet hip-width apart with knees slightly bent.
- Upright roller could be beside you, with palm of one hand resting lightly on top, if necessary, for balance.

Steps:
1. Bend a leg at the knee and lift the heel towards the buttocks, using your free hand to hold the leg at the ankle.
2. You should feel the stretch at the front of the thigh.
3. Hold the quads stretch for 20-30 seconds.
4. Repeat the quads stretch on the other leg, with your hand on the roller for support as necessary.

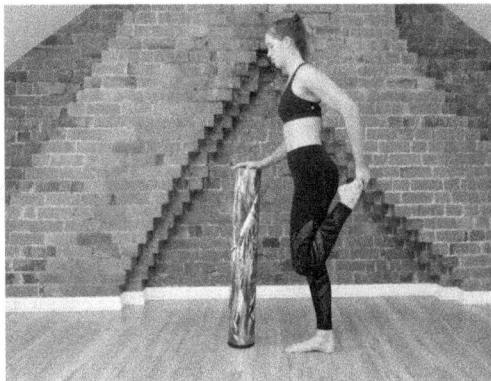

Tips:
- Keep the knee of the leg that you are standing on slightly bent throughout stretch.
- Try to keep weight into the heel of this foot as well, to help with balance.
- If you can't reach your ankle with your hand to hold the stretch, use a heavy resistance thera-band, or towel, looped around the ankle to assist.
- Take your thigh further behind you to increase the stretch but maintain a neutral lumbar spine.
- Keep your neck and shoulders relaxed throughout.
- Try a quads massage on the roller on the floor, especially post exercise.

LATS STRETCH WITH A ROLLER

This exercise targets the superficial latissimus dorsi (lats) muscle group; a large, broad, flat muscle on the back that connects the arm to the spine and the pelvis.

Set up:
- In standing, place an upright roller about an arm's length away.
- Have your feet and knees hip-width apart and knees slightly bent.

Steps:
1. Bend forward at the hips.
2. Keeping your arms straight, place your right palm over the end of the roller, then your left palm on top of your right hand.
3. Lower your head and upper body so that *your head remains between the upper arms* as you "hang" from the roller, feeling the stretch especially at the edge of the shoulders.
4. Hold for 20-30 seconds.

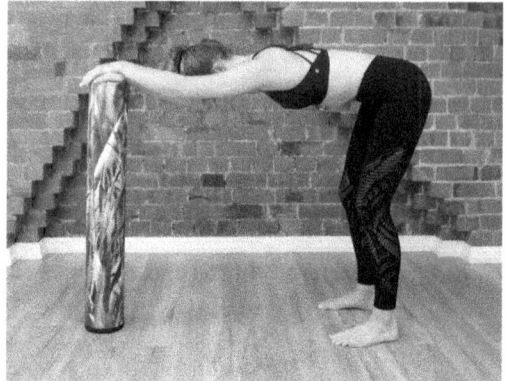

Tips:
- Aim for alignment horizontally through ears, shoulders and hips.
- You should also aim for vertical alignment with your lats stretch through the hips and ankles.
- Don't hold your breath. Ideally, use a deep breath in and then out to move further into your lats stretch.

Let it Roll

FROG STRETCH WITH A ROLLER

Frog stretch with a roller is similar to a "child's pose" in yoga. It helps to elongate the back and open up the hips, stretching the inner thighs and stretching the shoulders. You can also do the stretch without a roller.

Set up:
- In kneeling, place your roller horizontally on the floor in front of you.
- Place your wrists wide, on top of the roller, at each end, allowing the hands to flop over the roller.

Steps:

1. Put your feet together, knees apart.
2. Lower your buttocks towards your heels, letting your knees slide further apart.
3. Let your forehead rest on the floor and hands drop over the roller.
4. Hold for 30-60 seconds.

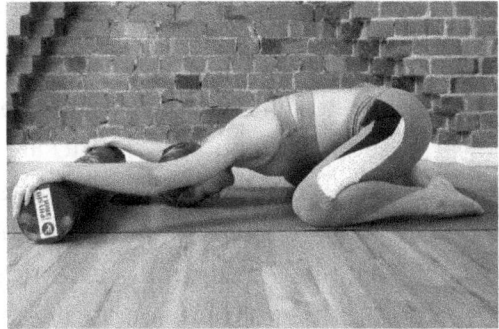

Tips:
- Just do the frog stretch in the range that is comfortable for you.
- There should be no knee pain, lower back pain or shoulder pain.
- Breathe throughout the stretch.
- If your knees are sore add a pillow under or behind the knee.

PASSIVE EXTENSIONS

Passive extensions are also known as "McKenzie" exercises. They are well known as the "go to" exercise if you have acute low back pain. Why? They help to restore your lumbar extension range and reduce muscle spasm.

Set up:
- Face down on the floor with arms bent, hands placed near the shoulders as shown.
- Feet are hip-width apart.

Steps:
1. Draw your shoulder blades down and back.
2. Breathe in and as you breathe out, push into your hands and lift your upper body off the floor, resting on your forearms or fully extending the elbows as shown (see tips).
3. Your hips and lower body stay on the floor (I like to think of hips as being "glued to the floor).
4. Breathe in as you lower.
5. Repeat x10.

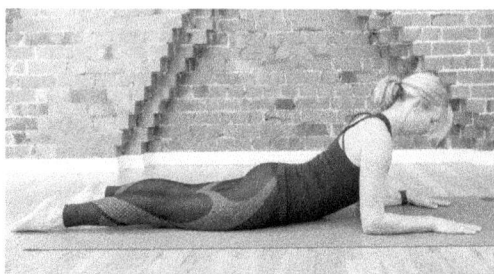

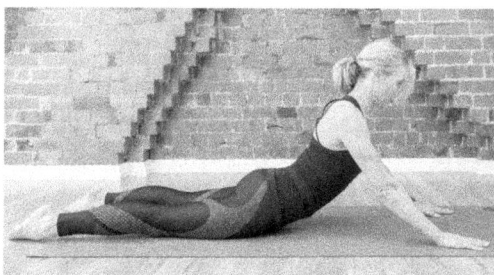

Tips:
- Don't push into pain. Stop short of it, and your range will improve over time.
- All backs differ in their flexibility – you may not fully extend your elbows but instead only get to your forearms or somewhere in between.
- Keep your bottom relaxed.
- Shoulders should not creep up to the ears.
- Tuck your chin a little.
- Do hourly (only x10 each time) as needed to settle acute back pain.

CHAPTER 8

Specific Roller Programs

A. Banish your back pain

Recent Sydney Uni research found that 7 out of 10 people with low back pain will have another episode of back pain within a year (4). It was shown that the only way to prevent this re-occurrence was with a prolonged exercise program, performed 2 to 3 days per week for 6 months or more.

The workout below fits the bill, combining flexibility and core exercises. It is designed to improve your hip and spine mobility and build strength in your core, quads and glute muscles. You will become more aware of your posture and alignment and how you are moving. This often results in you moving better and feeling better.

Remember that your back is strong and resilient, and exercise is medicine for backs.

Notes:

- This program assumes you have or are recovering from a low back pain episode.
- I suggest that you follow the order as listed.
- Read the instructions for each exercise thoroughly. Omit any exercises that aggravate your back pain, despite modification.
- Some exercises are without a roller initially as there are specifics about the exercise that should be mastered before introducing a roller.
- Once you are pain-free, progress the exercises by increasing the reps from x2 to x3 or substituting some of the harder options from the "Now You're on a Roll" section. Alternatively, try the "Benefit from the Basics" or the "Anything but Average" roller workouts on pages 188 and 190.

	REPS
1. Warm up in standing (page 43)	
2. Glutes with a roller (page 58)	both sides to fatigue
3. Wall push-up with a roller (page 56)	x10
4. Wall squat with roller, bicep curl (page 61)	x15
REPEAT X2-3 SETS	
5. Quads stretch (page 169)	20 sec hold
6. Abdominals – BKF +/- band at knees (page 48)	x15 each side
7. Abdominals – single knee lift (page 50)	x10 each leg
8. Star fish stretch (page 154)	20-30 seconds
REPEAT X2-3 SETS	
9. Abdominals hands overhead – one knee over hip (page 55)	x10 each leg
10. Bridging (no roller) (page 64)	x10
REPEAT X2-3 SETS	
11. Hip flexor stretch (page 155)	20-second hold
12. Leg stretches with a band (page 166)	hold each stretch 20-30 secs
13. Passive extensions (page 172)	x10
14. Windmill stretch (page 160)	x6-8 each side
15. Bird dog (page 72)	x3-5 reps
16. Frog stretch (page 171)	20-second hold

B. No more neck pain

There is evidence to suggest that you may reduce the risk of future neck discomfort by around 60% with an exercise program designed to improve neck strength and endurance (2).

The program below starts with some basic mobility exercises and awareness of head, neck and shoulders in space. This is a must, as often, if you experience neck pain, you first need to learn how to "let go" of tight, sore and overworked neck muscles. Then you can begin to strengthen the neck, shoulder and scapula muscles as well as improve core strength. A strong torso supports your head on top of your neck.

Notes:
- This program assumes you have or are recovering from neck pain.
- I suggest that you follow the order as listed.
- Read the instructions for each exercise thoroughly. Omit any exercises that aggravate your neck pain despite modification.
- Some exercises are without a roller initially as there are specifics about the exercise that should be mastered before introducing a roller.
- Triceps/flys/bench press (6, 7 and 8 below) can be done as a series with a starfish stretch in between sets.

	REPS
1. Warm up in standing (page 43)	
2. Head nod (page 77)	x10
3. Chin tuck (page 75)	x10
4. Wall push up with a roller (page 56)	x10
5. Roller reach and squeeze/ roller arm rotations (page 152)	x5 bilateral x5 unilateral
6. Triceps on a roller (page 108)	x10
7. Flys on a roller (page 110)	x10
8. Bench press on a roller (page 106)	x10
9. Starfish stretch (page 154)	x10

REPEAT X3 SETS

10. Thoracic roll out (page 157)	x30 seconds
11. Thoracic extension (page 158)	x4
12. Windmill stretch (page 160)	x6-8 each side
13. Hands overhead with roller (page 54)	x10 each side
14. Modified Biering-Sorenson (page 71)	x10
15. Basic bird dog (page 72)	x3 legs only
16. Frog stretch (page 171)	20-second hold

REPEAT X2 SETS

C. Lower limb legend

This workout targets quad and glute strength as well as your core. It will help with your balance and joint mobility and ease hip and knee pain to improve your day-to-day function.

Notes:
- I suggest that you follow the order as listed.
- Read the instructions for each exercise thoroughly. Omit any exercises that aggravate your knee pain (despite modification) for longer than 24 hours.
- Correct foot, knee and hip alignment are key components of this program.
- Some exercises are without a roller initially as there are specifics about the exercise that should be mastered before introducing a roller.

	REPS
1. Warm up in standing (page 43)	
2. Roller squat (page 80)	x20
3. Lunge with a roller – rotations (page 83)	x10 each side
4. Hip hinge/forward lean with a roller (page 66)	x15 each leg
REPEAT X2 SETS	
5. Glutes with a roller (page 58)	to fatigue
6. Basic wall squat with a roller (page 61)	x20
7. Roller hops (modified) (page 86)	x60 seconds
REPEAT X2-3 SETS	
8. Quads stretch (page 169)	x20 hold each side
9. Bent knee fallout with a band (page 48)	x10 each leg
10. Bridging on a roller with a band (page 95)	x15 each side
REPEAT X2-3 SETS	
11. Dead bug with a roller (page 100)	x10 each side
12. Bird dog (page 72)	x3-5 each side
REPEAT X2 SETS	
13. Leg stretches with a band (page 166)	20-second hold
14. Hip flexor stretch (page 155)	20-second hold
15. Quads massage with a roller (page 162)	30-60 seconds
16. ITB massage with a roller (page 164)	30-60 seconds each

D. Ultimate upper body

Training your upper body involves exercising your upper back, chest, shoulders, arms and core. Having a strong upper body reduces the risk of neck and shoulder pain. It will make lifting and overhead activities easier.

Notes:

- This program assumes you have minimal or no back or neck pain.
- Side plank is the hardest exercise. Do each side for 30-60 seconds.
- I suggest that you follow the order as listed.
- Read the instructions for each exercise thoroughly before you begin.

	REPS
1. Warm up (page 43)	
2. Wall push-up with a roller (page 56)	x10
3. Lunge with a roller – rotations (page 83)	x10 each side
4. Triceps push-up with a roller (page 92)	x10 each arm
5. Lats stretch with a roller (page 170)	20-second hold
6. Wall squats + band variations (page 61)	x20
REPEAT X2-3 SETS	
7. Roller reach and squeeze (page 152)	x5 bilateral
8. Shoulder circles (page 152)	x5 each side
9. Triceps on a roller (page 108)	x15
10. Flys on a roller (page 110)	x15
11. Bench press on a roller (page 106)	x15
12. Starfish stretch (page 154)	20-second hold
REPEAT X2-3 SETS	
13. Roller push-up (page 122)	x10
14. Frog stretch (page 171)	20 seconds
15. 4-point kneeling (page 112)	x3-5
REPEAT X2 SETS	
16. Side plank (page 142)	30-60 seconds each side
17. Thoracic roll out (page 157)	30-60 seconds
18. Windmill stretch (page 160)	x6-8 each side

E. Turbo charge your core

Your core is involved in everything that you do. Planks and push-ups are obvious core exercises because you have to contract your torso muscles to keep your spine from sagging. Some of the other exercises included in the program below are more subtle with their core activation.

Notes
- This is an advanced program and it assumes that you have no low back or neck pain.
- I suggest that you follow the order as listed.
- Read the instructions for each exercise thoroughly, especially the tips. Make the exercise easier if you find that you are using your back or neck muscles.

	REPS
1. Warm up in standing (page 43)	
2. Drinking bird (page 137)	x10 each leg
3. Lunge with a roller – rotations (page 83)	x10 each leg
4. Mountain climbers (page 130)	x10 each leg
REPEAT X3 SETS	
5. Roller jumps (page 125)	x30
6. Roller lunge with arm abduction + weight (page 127)	x20 each leg
REPEAT X2-3 SETS	
7. Single arm flys on a roller (page 111)	x15
8. Cross body push on a roller (page 107)	x15
9. Starfish stretch (page 154)	20-second hold
REPEAT X2-3 SETS	
10. Sit-ups a roller (page 102)	x20
11. Abdominals – single then double knee lift (page 105)	x10
12. Toe taps (page 144)	x10 each leg
REPEAT X2-3 SETS	
13. Hip flexor stretch (page 155)	x20 seconds each side
14. Roller plank (page 139)	60-second hold
15. Passive extensions (page 172)	x10
16. Bird dog on a roller (page 132)	x5
17. Windmill stretch (page 160)	x6-8
18. Frog stretch (page 171)	20-second hold

F. Boost your balance

The following exercises will all challenge and as such contribute to improving your balance. They progress from simple to advanced exercises with single stance positions and unstable stance positions (as anytime you make the surface underneath you smaller or less stable, you are going to have to use more balance!). There is also a focus on glutes and core strength.

Notes:
- This program assumes that you want (or need) to improve your balance (e.g. following an ankle injury or as you age). It is structured differently to the previous programs.
- Warm up first then with the balance exercise options choose either the A or B exercise that suits your ability. As you improve try the harder options.
- There are glutes and core strengthening exercises throughout this program.
- I suggest that you follow the order as listed.
- Read the instructions for each exercise thoroughly.

	REPS
1. Warm up (page 43)	
2. Glutes with a roller (page 58)	to fatigue
3. Step stance balance (page 69)	x3
4. A. Single leg balance and roll (page 70) **OR**	30-60 seconds
B. Roller balance (page 88)	
REPEAT X2 SETS	
5. Lunge with a roller – rotations (page 83)	x10-15
6. A. Single knee lift & tap (page 90) **OR**	x10-15
B. Single knee lift and lunge (page 91)	
REPEAT X2-3 SETS	
7. A. Roller hops/steps (page 86) **OR**	60 seconds
B. Roller jumps (page 125)	
8. A. Forward lean with a roller (page 66) **OR**	x10-15
B. Drinking bird (page 137)	
9. Wall squats with a roller (page 61)	x20-30
REPEAT X2 SETS	
10. Dead bug (page 100)	x20
11. Starfish stretch (page 154)	20 seconds
12. Advanced roller bridges (page 134)	x10
13. 4-point kneel (page 112)	x5
14. Leg stretches (page 166)	20-second hold each

CHAPTER 9

Graded Roller Programs

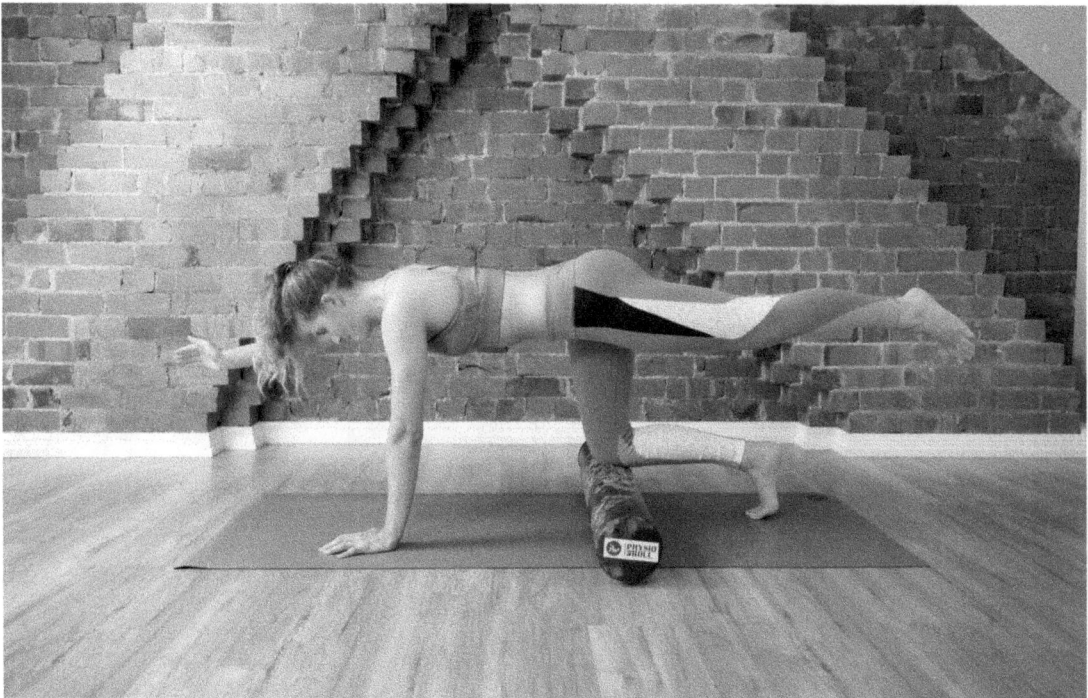

A. Benefit from the basics

- This workout assumes you have minimal pain.
- I suggest that you follow the order as listed.
- Read the instructions for each exercise thoroughly. Omit any exercises that are uncomfortable, despite modification.
- Some exercises are without a roller initially as there are specifics about the exercise that should be mastered before introducing a roller.

	REPS
1. Warm up in standing (page 43)	
2. Wall push-up with a roller (page 56)	x10
3. Glutes with a roller (page 58)	to fatigue one side, other side next set
4. Basic wall squat with a roller, theraband bicep curl (page 61)	x15-20
REPEAT X2 SETS	
5. Single knee lift and tap (page 90)	x10 each leg
6. Hip hinge with a roller forward lean (page 66)	x10 each leg
REPEAT X2-3 SETS	
7. Roller abdominals – hands overhead (page 54)	x10
8. Roller abdominals – hands overhead, static knee over hip (page 55)	x10 each leg
9. Roller abdominals – hands overhead, moving leg (page 55)	x10 each leg
REPEAT X2-3 SETS	
10. Hip flexor stretch (page 155)	20-second hold each leg
11. Bent knee fall out (with a band) (page 49)	x15 each side
12. Bridge on a roller (+/- a band) (page 95)	x10
REPEAT X2-3 SETS	
13. Starfish stretch (page 154)	20-second hold
14. Thoracic roll out (page 157)	30-60 seconds
15. Leg stretches (page 166)	20-30 seconds each
16. Basic bird dog (page 72)	legs only x5 each side
17. Frog stretch (page 171)	20-second hold

B. Anything but average

This is a mid-level program designed to challenge your core and balance and build strength. You have the opportunity to make any of the exercises easier or harder by reading the tips and suggestions in the main exercise section.

Notes:
- This workout assumes you have no or minimal pain.
- I suggest that you follow the order as listed.
- Read the instructions for each exercise thoroughly.

	REPS
1. Warm up in standing (page 43)	
2. Hip hinge with a roller forward lean (page 66)	x10 each leg
3. Lunge with a roller – rotations (page 83)	x10 each leg
4. Roller squat (page 80)	x20
REPEAT X2-3 SETS	
5. Wall push-up with a roller, on toes (page 56)	x10
6. Single knee lift and lunge (page 91)	x10 each leg
7. Roller hops (low impact) (page 86)	60 seconds
REPEAT X2-3 SETS	
8. Single arm flys on a roller (page 111)	x15 each side
9. Cross body pushes on a roller (page 107)	x10 each side
10. Starfish stretch (page 154)	20-second hold
REPEAT X2-3 SETS	
11. Abdominals – single knee then double knee lift (page 105)	x10 each side
12. Advanced abdominals – toe taps (page 144)	x5-10 each leg
13. Dead bug (page 100)	x10 each side
14. Hip flexor stretch (page 155)	20-second hold each leg
15. Roller plank on knees (page 116)	30-60 second hold
16. Passive extensions (page 172)	x10
17. 4-point kneeling (page 112)	arm & leg x3-5 each side
18. Frog stretch with a roller (page 171)	20-second hold

C. Roller challenge

This is an advanced roller routine that will work your entire body and challenge your core and balance.

Notes
- As an advanced program it is assumed that you are not experiencing any pain and have a high level of fitness.
- I suggest that you follow the order as listed.
- Read the instructions for each exercise thoroughly, especially the tips. Make the exercise easier if you find that you are using your back or neck muscles.

	REPS
1. Warm up in standing (page 43)	
2. Drinking bird (page 137)	x10 each leg
3. Roller lunges with weighted alternating lateral raise (page 128)	x20 each leg
4. Single knee lift to lunge (page 91)	x15 each leg
5. Mountain climbers (page 130)	x15 each leg
REPEAT X2-3 SETS	
6. Roller jumps (page 125)	x60 seconds
7. Push-up on a roller (at feet) (page 124)	x10 - 20
8. Advanced Roller Bridge (page 134)	x5-10 each leg
REPEAT X2-3 SETS	
9. Toe taps (page 144)	x10 each leg
10. Advanced abdominals – single leg lower (page 146)	x10 each leg
11. Star fish stretch (page 154)	20-second hold
REPEAT X2 SETS	
12. Side plank (page 142)	30-60 second hold each side
13. Passive extensions (page 172)	x10
14. Bird dog on a roller (page 132)	x3 each side, 30-second hold
15. Frog stretch with a roller (page 171)	20-second hold
16. Quads massage with a roller (page 162)	x30-60 seconds
17. Hip flexor stretch (page 155)	x20 seconds each side
18. Windmill stretch (page 160)	x6-8 each side

About the Author

Fiona has been passionate about exercise her entire life.

She was born and lived in Bowral in the beautiful NSW Southern Highlands until she finished secondary school. She walked to and from school each day (starting as a five-year-old) and played every team sport available. She cycled all over the district for hours on end and as a teenager developed a deep love of running.

At school she particularly enjoyed biology and her interest in sports and the human body led her to a physiotherapy degree at Sydney University.

She met her future husband, Roy, while working at Royal Prince Alfred Hospital in her first "intern" year out of university. He encouraged her to travel before they married and so she headed off on a "gap year" to the UK, using her physio skills to work as a locum in three British hospitals which was accented with backpacking trips across Europe.

Fiona returned to Australia to marry, begin working in private practice and then establish her own successful private practice in Sans Souci, in Southern Sydney. She introduced Pilates (a relatively new concept in Australia back then) into her practice in 1997 and then discovered that she was expecting twins.

Having two small babies to look after, as well as (at that time) a sick husband and two small businesses (her husband had his own small business as well) meant something had to give. She reluctantly sold the practice but continued to work part time in private physiotherapy practices in the inner west, St George and Sutherland Shire. Exercise still featured heavily in her life, mostly as a way of keeping fit and healthy (and sane!).

Fast forward to 2008 when Fiona's husband unfortunately and unexpectedly passed away.

Exercise suddenly became her therapy as well as a way to keep fit. The happy hormones that the brain releases (mostly serotonin) during exercise helped her to cope with the enormous loss of her husband and the huge task of bringing up three young children (then aged six, nine and nine) without their dad.

She began working at a physiotherapy practice in Sydney's eastern Suburbs three months after her husband's death. Teaching small group exercise classes was a "safe" way for Fiona to interact with people again as she found it far less intimidating and less personal than a one-on-one client interaction (she still has some of those original clients in her classes today!). She was basically instructing core motor control and teaching those who had injured their backs or necks how to move well again with safety and confidence.

Over the years these classes evolved, closely following the latest evidence-based research to include elements of Pilates, yoga, weight training and physiotherapy.

Fiona designs, teaches and supervises both individual and small group exercise programs. Her clients include athletes, chronic pain sufferers, cancer survivors and people post-surgery, as well as individuals with osteoporosis, back and neck pain, knee, hip and shoulder pain, and kids.

Her clients want to ease their pain and improve their flexibility. Her aim is to use exercise as medicine, to help them to increase their muscle strength, core motor control and mobility. To help them to improve their balance, proprioception and posture. She is also a big believer in functional exercises. It may be great to have toned arms and a nice rounded bottom, but it is even better to know that you can use those attributes to safely lift your child or grandchild off the floor without doing your back in!

The long foam roller has become her exercise tool of choice, simply because it promotes the ability to gain strength, awareness and conditioning just by balancing on it or with it. It is accessible by all populations whether young, old, beginner or advanced. It can be used on its own or with weights or resistance bands.

Fiona's love of exercise over the years has kept her strong, sane and healthy. She practices what she preaches. It also fostered a love of exercise in her children.

In 2012, an old high school flame re-entered her life and they married in 2015. Later that year she successfully climbed Mt Kilimanjaro for the charity Cure Cancer and has continued to hike and bike through the UK, NZ, Vietnam, Yosemite and all over Australia.

To date she has completed 25 City to Surfs, 12 half-marathons and she proudly ran the New York Marathon, in 2016 (at the age of 48) in a respectable four hours and four minutes beating her then 18-year-old twin sons by 30 and 55 mins respectively – she never misses a chance to remind them!!

Today, Fiona continues to work part-time in a Double Bay physiotherapy practice, and she consults privately and teaches online courses and group classes via her *Physio on a Roll* website.

Fiona is an accreditated GLAD Australia Physiotherapist, and a Pinc and Steel and DMA Pilates-trained practioner.

Along with husband Chris, she believes exercise is medicine. They are both passionate about leading by example and run, cycle, walk and paddle socially in a dragon boat. They lift weights and of course use a foam roller. Both exercise to stay fit and healthy and because they like the way it makes them feel, knowing that it will allow them to age well.

Fiona Naayen
B.App.Sc.Physio A.P.A.M.
fiona@physioonaroll.com.au
www.physioonaroll.com.au

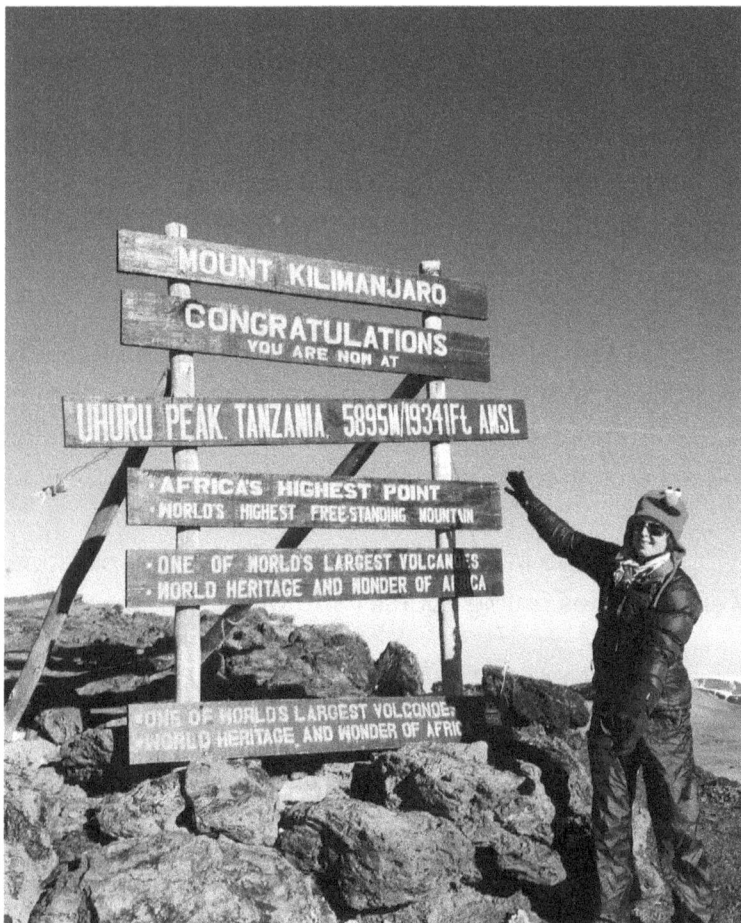

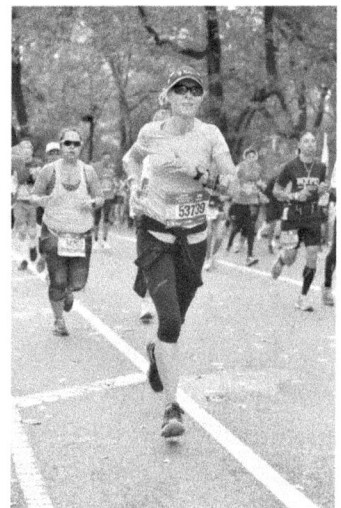

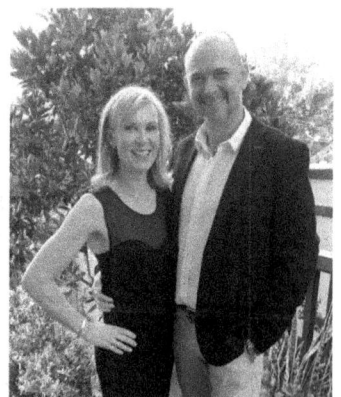

Let it Roll

Afterword

Firstly, congratulations! By reading through *Let it Roll* you will have gained an understanding of how exercise can be used to manage pain, improve strength and mobility and help you move and function better. Often when we understand how and why something benefits us, we are more likely to do it!

You should also have a new-found appreciation for your foam roller and its myriad of uses and benefits – understanding how to incorporate it into existing exercises to activate and strengthen your core, challenge your balance and "let go" of tight muscles, especially the muscles in your neck and shoulders.

Please don't feel compelled to do every exercise in this book, or in each section. Hopefully there are many exercises that have resonated with you that you will continue to incorporate into your daily routine or each workout. And don't forget to use this book as a reference when that back or shoulder niggle flares up.

If you are someone who is experiencing pain, please take your time with the exercises. A consistent approach works best and it can take 3-6 months before you see results. Start without a roller if necessary and visit the *Physio on a Roll* website for more tips on basic exercises. Also don't assume that everybody wants or indeed needs to do the "high roller" exercises. By working through the book you will also have gained an appreciation of how to adjust exercises to make them easier or harder to suit your particular issues.

If you are an experienced exerciser, a "now you're on a roll" or a "high roller" and are after more variety in workouts or exercises also head to the *Physio on a Roll* website. There are many more exercises and routines, plenty with Swiss balls and resistance bands that are not included in this book.

Above all, I hope your roller does not languish in the corner but takes pride of place in the lounge room or gym where you can use it daily.

Offers

Roller

Purchase your very own Physio on a Roll custom designed roller (as featured throughout *Let it Roll*).

90cm in length with a 15cm diameter, made from high quality, high density 35+ EVA foam. Lightweight and portable, Physio on a Roll rollers are very firm and will not collapse, distort or dent.

Designed for long-term use, the decorative PV cover ensures that the rollers surface is durable, won't absorb fluids or dirt and easily wipes clean.

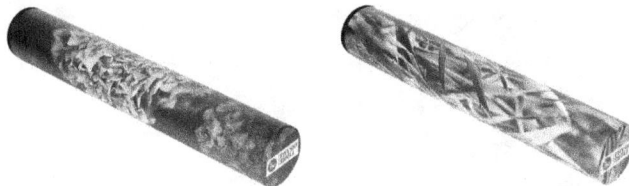

30% discount for *Let it Roll* purchasers = $33 (normally $47) + $15 postage and handling (Australia only)

Use code LIRBook https://physioonaroll.com.au/our-shop/

One-on-One Consultation

50% off a 60-minute one-on-one live online consultation with author
Fiona Naayen B.App.Sc. Physio A.P.A.M.
This is your chance to have a personal consultation with the author of *Let it Roll*.
Delivered via zoom, your live telehealth consultation will include:
- a pre-appointment questionnaire.
- 60-minute live discussion with Fiona who will listen to your history, concerns and goals, conduct an online assessment and then with you, devise an exercise program that suits you personally.
- a personalised exercise plan with detailed photos and videos delivered via email after the recorded zoom call with follow up text and email support.

Value $500
Let it Roll offer = $250.

Contact fiona@physioonaroll.com.au and quote "book consult" for more details or to take up the offer.

Banish your Back Pain Course

10-week online group class "Banish your Back Pain", $1390 valued at $1690.

A comprehensive online program that teaches you how to manage your back pain and build strength so that you move better, feel better and live better.

Includes:
- pre-appointment questionnaire.
- a 45-minute live one-on-one consultation to assess your problems.
- 1 live 45 minute group exercise class each week (maximum number = 8/ class), 3 sessions times to choose from.
- 2 recorded 45 minute classes/week, delivered to your inbox and performed in your own time.

- text and email support.
- weekly education sessions delivered to your inbox to address the habits that may be adding to your back pain.

Contact fiona@physioonaroll.com.au quoting "banish your back pain course" to register interest or if you would like more details. Payment plans are available.

*Subscribe to our fortnightly email and receive the code to unluck our exclusive exercises at Physio on a Roll: www.physioonaroll.com.au

Like us on **Instagram** @physioonaroll and **Facebook,** where we share our latest news and post-exercise tips and insights.

References

1. Foam Rolling and Muscle and Joint Proprioception After Exercise-Induced Muscle Damage J Athl Train 2020 Jan; 55(1):58-64.

2. Foam Rolling for Delayed-Onset Muscle Soreness and Recovery of Dynamic Performance Measures. J Athl Train. 2015 Jan; 50(1):5–13.

3. De Campos et al (2018) Exercise programs may be effective in preventing a new episode of neck pain: a systematic review and meta-analysis. Journal of Physiotherapy 64 (3) 159-165.

4. Ferreira et al (2020) People considering exercise to prevent low back pain recurrence prefer exercise programs that differ from programs known to be effective: a discrete choice experiment. Journal of Physiotherapy Volume 66, Issue 4, 10, 249-255.

5. La Trobe University.

6. Sherrington et al. Exercise for preventing falls in older people living in the community. Cochrane Database of Systematic Reviews 2019, Issue 1.

7. "Balance Yourself" by Next Step Allied Health 2017.

8. Shubert,T.E.(2011) Evidence-based exercise prescription for balance and falls prevention: a current review of the literature. Journal of geriatric physical therapy, 34(3), 100-108

9. Schoenfeld et al Differential effects of attentional focus strategies during long-term resistance training. March 2018. European Journal of Sport Science 18(5):1-8

10. Idorn M, Thor Straten P. Exercise and cancer: from "healthy" to "therapeutic"? Cancer Immunol Immunother. 2017 May; 66(5):667-671.

11. Beck BR, Daly RM, Fiatarone-Singh MA, Taaffe DR: Exercise and Sports Science Australia (ESSA) position statement on exercise prescription for the prevention and management of osteoporosis. J Science Med Sport 20(5):438-445, May 2017

12. Bunzli S, Smith A, Schütze R, Lin I, O'Sullivan P. Making Sense of Low Back Pain and Pain-Related Fear. J Orthop Sports Phys Ther. 2017 Sep; 47(9):628-636.

13. Dr. Jarod Hall d.p.t

14. http://blogs.bmj.com/bjsm/2016/02/23/train-for-life-exercise-is-medicine

15. Valenzuela et al (2020) Hippocampal plasticity underpins long term gains from resistance exercise in MCI. Neuroimage: clinical 25.

16. "The New Rules of Lifting for Life" Lou Schuler and Alwyn Cosgrove

17. Sherrington et al (2016) Exercise to prevent falls in older adults: an updated systematic review and meta-analysis. British Journal of Sports Medicine.

18. Bricca et al (2019) Impact of exercise on articular cartilage in people at risk of, or with established, knee osteoarthritis: a systematic review of randomised controlled trials. British Journal of Sports Medicine 2019;**53:**940-947.

19. Glad Australia 2020.

20. Exercise is Medicine website-osteoporosis

21. Schmidt H, Bashkuev M, Weerts J, Graichen F, Altenscheidt J, Maier C, Reitmaier S. How do we stand? Variations during repeated standing phases of asymptomatic subjects and low back pain patients. J Biomech. 2018 Mar 21;70:67-76.

22. "Sit up straight" Time to re-evaluate. Slater et al. JOSPT 49(8)

23. Gerritsen RJS, Band GPH. Breath of Life: The Respiratory Vagal Stimulation Model of Contemplative Activity. Front Hum Neurosci. 2018 Oct 9; 12:3 97.

24. An update of stabilisation exercises for low back pain: A systematic review with meta-analysis. December 2014. BMC Musculoskeletal Disorders 15(1):416

25. Greg Dea and Rod Harris: Core Stability and Core Strength Are Not the Same. On Target publications

26. Parr, M., Price, P. D., & Cleather, D. J. (2017). Effect of a gluteal activation warm-up on explosive exercise performance. BMJ Open Sport & Exercise Medicine

27. Watson SL, Weeks BK, Weis L, Horan SA, and Beck BR: High Intensity Resistance and Impact Training Improves Bone Mineral Density and Physical Function in Postmenopausal Women With Osteopenia and Osteoporosis: The LIFTMOR Randomized Controlled Trial. J Bone Miner Res, Online Oct 2017.

28. Influence of Foam Rolling on Recovery From Exercise-Induced Muscle Damage J Strength Cond Res 2019 Sep; 33(9):2443-2452.

29. http://exerciseismedicine.com.au/wp-content/uploads/2020/04/EIM-FactSheet_General-Cancer_Professionals-2020.pdf

30. Osteoporosis Australia

31. http://www.pain-ed.com/wp-content/uploads/2014/02/Osullivan-and-Lin-Pain-management-today-2014.pdf

32. Nolan D, O'Sullivan K, Newton C, Singh G, Smith BE. Are there differences in lifting technique between those with and without low back pain? A systematic review. Scand J Pain. 2020 Apr 28; 20(2):215-227.

33. The myth of core stability by Professor Eyal Lederman

34. Greg Lehman www.trustme-Ed.com

35. Dr.Samspinelli

36. hamishthephysio

37. Comparison of Core Muscle Activation between a Prone Bridge and 6-RM Back Squats. Tillaar J Human Kinetics. 2018 Jun 13;62:43-53.

38. webMD

39. www.healthline.com

40. physiopedia

41. "Strong" Lou Schuler and Alwyn Cosgrove

42. "Back Mechanic" Stuart McGill

43. The Training Effects of Foam Rolling on Core Strength Endurance, Balance, Muscle Performance and Range of Motion: A Randomized Controlled Trial. J Sports Sci Med. 2019 Jun 1;18(2):229-238.

44. Nolan D, O'Sullivan K, Newton C, Singh G, Smith BE. Are there differences in lifting technique between those with and without low back pain? A systematic review. Scand J Pain. 2020 Apr 28;20(2):215-227.

45. Evan Osar: Low back pain – the myth of the weak core – part 1 OTP books.com

46. Evan Osar: Low back pain – the myth of the weak core – part 2 OTP books.com

47. Xiao et al Front Psychol. 2017; 8: 874. The Effect of Diaphragmatic Breathing on Attention, Negative Affect and Stress in Healthy Adults

Acknowledgements

I would like to say a huge thank you to all my clients who believed in this project from the very start. Your enthusiasm for my teaching methods and my need to justify and explain everything has been an inspiration. I am grateful for your daily support – encouraging me, laughing with me, giving me ideas and trying out new exercises.

Thank you to my sons, Thomas and William, who were the early models for the exercises on my website Physio on a Roll. My daughter, Samantha, is the model in most of the photos featured throughout this book and I am extremely grateful for her support, athletic ability and patience.

My final thanks is to both of my husbands, Roy and Chris. I am extraordinarily lucky to have been supported by two men who have believed in me and backed me unreservedly throughout my physiotherapy career. Chris (fondly known by all as "Orf"), you are my number one fan, my foundation, and an eternal optimist. Always positive, you have been with me every step of the way with the development of my website and now this book. You have cheered me on, motivated me and loved me. I am eternally grateful that you crashed back into my life.

Glossary

Diaphragm – dome-shaped skeletal muscle that separates the chest from the abdomen and assists with breathing.

Supine – lying on your back.

Prone – lying on your stomach.

Vertigo – dizziness associated with inner ear problems.

Sarcopenia – age related muscle loss.

Glutes – buttock muscles. Consists of gluteus medius, gluteus maximus and gluteus minimus.

Lats – latissimus dorsi, surface back muscle group that connects the upper arm to the torso.

Scapula – shoulder blade.

Quadratus lumborum – muscle in the lumbar spine that attaches to every vertebra. It helps to stabilise the spine.

Oblique muscles – the external and internal oblique muscles are layered with the **transversus abdominus** to form the abdominal wall. They enable twisting motions and add to core stability.

Rectus abdominus – the "six pack" muscle at the front of the abdomen.

Cervical spine – neck.

Thoracic spine – longest part of your spine, connecting your neck to your lower back. Ribs attach to it.

Lumbar spine – lower back.

Neutral spine – shape of the normal spine when standing upright; position of the spine where it is the most relaxed and free of tension.

Proprioception – awareness of the position of your body in space.

Protraction – shoulder blades moving away from the spine.

Retraction – shoulder blades moving towards the spine.

Scaption – straight arm lifting out from the body at a 45-degree angle.

Pilates – a method of exercise that consists of low impact movements that aim to improve muscular strength and endurance.

Clinical Pilates – a unique approach that "distills" the pilates exercise repertoire into a clinical package that is integrated with the broad knowledge base of physiotherapists.

DMA – Dance Medicine Australia, Clinical Pilates Training that uses a movement-based classification and treatment approach.

GLAD – an exercise and rehabilitation program developed by researchers in Denmark for people with hip and knee pain that has been clinically proven to decrease pain and improve function.

Pinc and Steel – cancer rehabilitation programs run by trained physiotherapists.

Notes

Let it Roll